THE MENOPAUSE ANSWER BOOK

Treatments & Solutions for Your Unique Symptoms

MARSHA LYNN SPELLER, MD

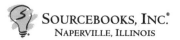
SOURCEBOOKS, INC.®
NAPERVILLE, ILLINOIS

This book is not intended as a substitute for medical advice from a qualified physician. The intent of this book is to provide accurate general information in regard to the subject matter covered. If medical advice or other expert help is needed, the services of an appropriate medical professional should be sought.

Published by Sourcebooks, Inc.
P.O. Box 4410, Naperville, Illinois 60567-4410
(630) 961-3900
FAX: (630) 961-2168
www.sourcebooks.com

Library of Congress Cataloging-in-Publication Data
Speller, Marsha Lynn.
The menopause answer book: treatments and solutions for your unique symptoms
/ by Marsha Lynn Speller.
p. cm.
Includes bibliographical references and index.
ISBN 1-4022-0259-8 (alk. paper)
1. Menopause—Popular works. 2. Middle aged women—Health and hygiene—Popular works. I. Title.
RG186.S699 2004
618.1'75—dc22
2004001037

ISBN 1-4022-0259-8

Printed and bound in the United States of America
BG   10   9   8   7   6   5   4   3   2   1

To Lauren,
I want you to know everything
I'm learning about being a woman,
and
To John,
I want to help you understand us.
With love,
Mom

Acknowledgments

I want to acknowledge my husband Wes, my daughter Laurie, Pat Thomas, Calva Queenan, Lynn Kirby, Colleen Buchanan, and Deborah Werksman for their help and advice.

Table of Contents

Introduction

Millions of women reach middle age every year. The health risks of feminine midlife directly impact us, our families, our friends, and our employers. A failure to understand and anticipate our risks accounts for many of the health problems women are encountering as they age.

Good health and vitality depend on what we do to prevent problems as we age. A good health program can be developed at any age if we have information. My goal is to help you become an informed health-care consumer.

If you are struggling with medical problems, the advice in these pages can help stabilize your conditions as well as help you and your doctor better manage your illness.

Why did I get interested in this aspect of women's health?

My specialty is psychiatry, which gives me an experienced advantage. Psychiatry is predominantly the study of women across the life cycle: all of the major psychiatric symptoms are many times more common in women than in men.

Most women approach menopause with a positive outlook. We've paid attention to our health and have gotten regular check-ups and kept up with routine screenings. But many of us haven't been paying much attention to the symptoms of perimenopause, which are the first signals that change—physical and emotional— is coming. In my practice, I frequently see perimenopausal women who are experiencing early signs of future disease.

My husband calls my perimenopause "the fabulous 50s," although he's being sarcastic. In spite of all I knew about health in midlife, havoc broke out concerning my own health. I had more physical problems and symptoms at this time of my life than during the rest of my whole life put together. These symptoms disrupted my functioning. So I decided that I wanted to learn about the change of life, share my knowledge about this universal female phenomenon with other women, and teach them how to handle it.

This is a workbook, designed to help you assess yourself physically and emotionally during perimenopause, menopause, and postmenopause. Like my small group seminar, named "Change of Life," its purpose is to get you to interact with the presented material and examine how it may or may not apply to you. This book may help you clarify which midlife issues are relevant to you. As I wrote, I imagined myself talking with you face-to-face in one of my groups, answering your questions and exchanging ideas. This book isn't meant to be a substitute for medical evaluation, but it might be an adjunct to a meaningful discussion with your doctor.

There is so much good information out there that we are flooded with it, can't absorb it all, and have difficulty trying to figure out which information is personally relevant. Hence, I have included questions, screening tools, and fill-in charts. I've tried to be comprehensive and helpful in focusing on those issues that are personally relevant to you. I've also tried to help you formulate good questions for your doctors, and I'm encouraging you to design your own health plan. And for those of you who have already logged in many hours researching and reading on your own, I hope this book can help you collate your research into one useful reference that's all about you.

The Menopause Action Plan, or MAP, is a questionnaire designed as a summary self-assessment that should accompany your midlife physical examination, but often doesn't. It is personal and private;

you can choose to share your thoughts with your doctor or not. But it's your doctor who can best help you, if you are willing to talk about your problems, experiences, and concerns. Your MAP can help focus that discussion.

Most women I know approach this phase of their lives with trepidation and fear. The physical changes at this time of life are unwanted, and aging looms just around the corner. I believe that the more you know about yourself and how your body works, the more confidence you'll have and the more active a role you'll take in your own health care.

Hopefully, this book will have everything you need to know about managing your menopause and future health and will help you make your quiet commitment to change the things you must.

Here's to your good health,
Marsha Lynn Speller, MD

Part I

How Hormones Work

Chapter 1

Getting Personal about Menopause

Hot Flashes

The heat creeps up my neck into my hairline and sweat trickles down my back. It wakes me up at night, every night. I throw off my covers (while my husband has learned to anchor his side down with both arms straight and extended). First the quilt, then the blanket, then the sheet, four or five times a night; off, on, off, on. So, by 6 A.M., I'm ready for a nap. My husband says I flash 'til I crash. My solution: fans, lots of them. I cradle their remote controls in my sleep and flip them off and on throughout the night. I'll beat this heat yet.

Forgetfulness

As I was making microwave sausage, I decided to start the car to warm it up. I locked myself out of the house and tried to use my car phone to call my husband, who was in bed upstairs. But I couldn't remember our new phone number, so I broke in through the back door. I finished making breakfast and ate it. Then, I went upstairs to dress for work. When I came back down, you guessed it—I was out of gas. I had forgotten I left the car engine running. Early Alzheimer's? No. CRS (Can't Remember Stuff).

Moodiness

Little things just set me off. I guess I've gotten short-tempered and impatient. I'm always criticizing everyone at home about every-thing. I need to shut up and bite my tongue, but the pressure to blurt out some sarcastic remark is just too great. Well, my husband and kids finally asked for a temporary separation during which I get to live at the office and come home for showers, a change of clothes, and (these are their terms) some Prozac. Now that's pressure...

Sex

It's not often that both our kids are out of the house and my hus-band and I are alone (and awake at the same time). He'll get that cute little smile and a twinkle in his eye, and we both say, "Yeah...." My heart is going thump, thump and I'm feeling warm and affec-tionate with him. Then, nothing. Dry as the Sahara. So I take out my shopping bag full of five herbal blends, four lubricating gels, three French creams, two soothing lotions, and a pint of petroleum jelly and, finally, we work it out. Somehow, it just doesn't seem the same...

Weight Gain

I look in the mirror and who do I see? A middle-aged woman who stares back at me. She looks suspiciously like my mother. And when I stand up and look down at my feet, the view is obstructed. You, too? Let's meet. I think if we talk we'll find ways to fight the flashes, the moods, and the cellulite.

So listen, ladies. Here it is; this is what we need:

- Something that will explain all of this and explain it more than once and keep it simple;

- Something to help kick the hormone habit—we can't take hormone replacements forever;
- Something to help us eat smart (without giving up chocolate);
- Something to help us with exercise (yes, we need it, and yes, it's supposed to feel that way);
- Something to help us get our problems and needs across to our doctors;
- And the answer to the question on everyone's mind: will these symptoms ever go away or am I headed for divorce?

We need a menopause map.

Chapter 2

In the Beginning...

Femaleness is the result of hormones, specifically, of estrogen. We are females because our bodies produce much higher levels of estrogen than males do.

Estrogen comes from our ovaries where our eggs are produced. We are born with about two million egg follicles (egg sacs) in our ovaries and, by our first period (sometime during puberty), we have four hundred to five hundred thousand follicles left. Egg follicles are fragile, susceptible to disintegration, injury, malnourishment, and loss. We lose about one thousand a month. But since we only ovulate four to five hundred times during our childbearing years, we have enough left to produce children.

Estrogen is important to a woman's health and plays an important role in every phase of her life because it exerts its influence across the life span.

During puberty, estrogen is responsible for our physical and emotional characteristics. During the young adult years, estrogen is responsible for our fertility. Throughout our lives, estrogen supports our immune system, protecting us from stress, from the effects of bad habits, and from disease. By the time we reach thirty-five, our estrogen levels have begun to decline and subtle changes start to occur in our bodies. In our mature years, the change in estrogen production combines with risks for disease and has an enormous influence over our future health. And, unlike the women who came before us, we are living thirty to forty years beyond menopause.

In the last 150 years, our life span has doubled. We will encounter many health issues throughout this long life.

A woman's life span can be divided into four "seasons" — puberty, young adulthood, midlife, and maturity. For all women, hormonal output will change as time passes.

Puberty is a time when estrogen production in our bodies surges forward, sometimes unevenly. This is evidenced by the appearance of our sexual characteristics: pubic hair, breasts, a period, and fertility.

We have high levels of estrogen in our bodies during the young-adult years. The life peak of estrogen production is reached when we are twenty-eight years old. The ovaries, which make estrogen, are endocrine organs; they produce hormones in sync with other hormone-producing glands, i.e., the pituitary, thyroid, thymus, and adrenal glands. Estrogen, like the hormones produced from the other glands, is protective and helps us weather sustained periods of stress. The high levels of estrogen present during the young-adult years can mask the long-term effects of the bad habits we acquire (such as overeating, drinking, failure to exercise, eating poor-quality food, and smoking). Basically, it is estrogen that keeps us healthy when our health habits are not good.

Emotional health depends on estrogen, also. After the onset of puberty, all the major psychiatric disorders become more common in women than in men. This difference between men and women is due to our hormones.

At midlife, we experience the symptoms of perimenopause, that roller-coaster ride of physical and mental symptoms that occur as our estrogen levels fall and before our period actually stops.

When menopause finally occurs, many of us treat it like an uninvited guest because it is the sign of our aging and the beginning of our maturity. In our mature years, estrogen production changes: our ovaries produce less estrogen and our bodies utilize a different mechanism to produce a less potent form of estrogen. When combined with our risks for disease at this age, the impact on our future health is significant.

Chapter 3

The Normal Menstrual Cycle

Just what is the menstrual cycle? For many women, menstruation governs much of daily life. We have accustomed ourselves to an emerging cycle with its ebb and flow of physical and psychological effects, and have learned to plan our activities around our periods.

The hormones that choreograph the menstrual cycle are:

- Gonadotropin-releasing hormone (GnRH), which is found in the brain area known as the hypothalamus
- Follicle-stimulating hormone (FSH)
- Luteinizing hormone (LH), which is secreted by the pituitary gland in the brain
- Estrogen and progesterone, which are made in the ovaries and secreted to the uterus (the target tissue, where menstrual blood flow results)

The following figure graphs the menstrual cycle with its corresponding hormonal and biological changes.

A menstrual cycle consists of four phases that a woman goes through every month (every lunar month, averaging twenty-eight days).

The first phase of the menstrual cycle is the *menstrual phase*, which begins with the first day of bleeding and lasts from one to

Changes During the Menstrual Cycle

A menstrual cycle is regulated by the complex interaction of hormones: luteinizing hormone and follicle-stimulating hormone, which are produced by the pituitary gland, and the female sex hormones estrogen and progesterone, which are produced by the ovaries.

The menstrual cycle begins with menstrual bleeding (menstruation), which marks the first day of the follicular phase. Bleeding occurs when levels of estrogen and progesterone decrease, causing the thickened lining of the uterus (endometrium) to degenerate and be shed. During the first half of this phase, the follicle-stimulating hormone level increases slightly, stimulating the development of several follicles. Each follicle contains an egg. Later, as the follicle-stimulating hormone level decreases, only one follicle continues to develop. This follicle produces estrogen.

The ovulatory phase begins with a surge in luteinizing hormone and follicle-stimulating hormone levels. Luteinizing hormone stimulates egg release (ovulation), which usually occurs 16 to 32 hours after the surge begins. The estrogen level peaks during the surge, and the progesterone level starts to increase.

During the luteal phase, levels of luteinizing hormone and follicle-stimulating hormone decrease. The ruptured follicle closes after releasing the egg and forms a corpus luteum, which produces progesterone. Later in this phase, the level of estrogen increases. Progesterone and estrogen cause the lining of the uterus to thicken more. If the egg is not fertilized, the corpus luteum degenerates and no longer produces progesterone, the estrogen level decreases, the lining degenerates and is shed, and a new menstrual cycle begins.

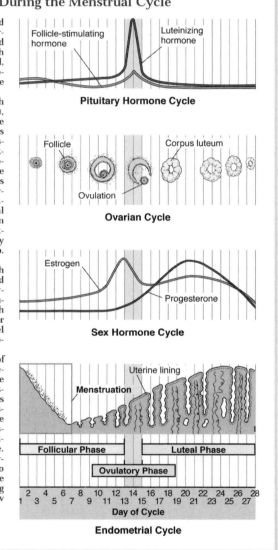

From the *Merck Manual of Medical Information – Second Home Edition*, p. 1347, edited by Mark H. Beers. Copyright 2003 by Merck & Co., Inc., Whitehouse Station, NJ.

five days. It is the sloughing off of the uterine lining. Both progesterone and estrogen are at their lowest points during this phase.

The second phase, the *follicular* or *postmenstrual phase*, begins approximately on day six. It is the most variable phase and can last five to ten days, depending on the length of a woman's cycle. During this phase, the hypothalamus generates gonadotropin-releasing hormone (GnRH) and the pituitary generates follicle-stimulating hormone (FSH), which stimulate cells within the ovaries, called follicles, to grow an egg. Luteinizing hormone (LH) is also produced, and this stimulates the egg follicle to produce estrogen. During this phase, estrogen levels are rising.

The third phase of the menstrual cycle, the *ovulatory phase*, lasts about two days. During this phase, the egg ruptures from the follicle under the stimulation of the pituitary's luteinizing hormone (LH). This mature egg is released into the fallopian tube and the remainder of the ruptured follicle develops into the *corpus luteum*, which produces high levels of estrogen and progesterone.

The fourth and final phase of the menstrual cycle, the *luteal* or *premenstrual phase*, lasts about fourteen days. If the egg is not fertilized within twenty-four hours of its release, progesterone production falls. After eleven to fourteen days, the blood supply to the uterine wall diminishes and the lining begins to slough off, so menstruation (blood flow) begins again.

The Four Phases of the Menstrual Cycle

I. The Menstrual Phase — lasts 1–5 days
   Symptoms: Menstrual bleeding (your 1st day)
                 Bloating
                 Cramping
                 Tiredness
                 Back Pain

II. The Follicular (or Postmenstrual) Phase — lasts 5–10 days
   Symptoms: Energetic
                 Confident
                 Sexy

III. The Ovulatory Phase — lasts 2 days
   Symptoms: Occasional brief back pain when the egg ruptures
                 from its sac.
   You are your most fertile at this time; plan ahead.

IV. The Luteal (or Premenstrual) Phase — lasts 14 days
   Symptoms: Irritability
                 Bloating
                 Anger
                 Depression
                 In short, the infamous PMS symptoms

The Average Cycle

Day	1-6	6-12	12-14	14-28
Phase	I	II	III	IV

MY CYCLE

Keep a calendar for three consecutive months to record the days of each phase.

Month 1:

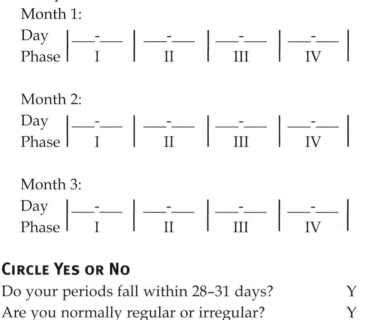

Day
Phase I   II   III   IV

Month 2:

Day
Phase I   II   III   IV

Month 3:

Day
Phase I   II   III   IV

CIRCLE YES OR NO

Do your periods fall within 28–31 days?   Y   N
Are you normally regular or irregular?   Y   N
Do you have PMS symptoms during Phase IV?   Y   N
If so, which ones?   _____

_____

_____

_____

PMS can continue all the way through to menopause, and it often intensifies perimenopausal symptoms.

During perimenopause and until menopause (the complete cessation of your normal menstrual cycle), the cardinal sign of the change of life is change in your menstrual cycle, its rhythm and its flow. Subtle changes actually occur much earlier than you expect, starting in our mid-thirties. On the not-so-subtle side, if you have PMS, it usually gets worse during the perimenopause years so that you can experience an intense mix of both PMS and perimenopause symptoms.

Estrogen production and flow changes twice during our life span: during puberty and during perimenopause. In fact, I sometimes think of perimenopause as a kind of midlife reversal of adolescence. Susan Love, MD, has beautifully described these changes as a hormonal dance.[1]

Quiz

At what age did you have your first period? _____

How long did it take your periods to finally
    become regular? _____

If you are perimenopausal, when do you think your
    symptoms started? _____

Are they getting more intense? _____

If you are postmenopausal, when do you estimate you
    had your last period? _____

How many years has it been since your last period? _____

Chapter 4

The Power of Estrogen

What's happening to my body?

Inevitably, for all of us, hormonal output changes as time passes. Males change in a steady, slow fashion with progressive hormonal decline. Females are rhythmic, and the midlife transition can be abrupt and jarring when that rhythm is disrupted. The only change comparable is puberty, when that rhythm began. Estrogen and progesterone are the female hormones that regulate change, and estrogen is the more influential. The life peak of estrogen production is reached by age twenty-eight (which coincides with our peak bone mass). Estrogen levels then plateau until age thirty-five, when they begin their linear decline. Midlife is just around the corner and the early, baffling signs of perimenopause begin. In America alone, thirty-one million women were born between 1946 and 1964 (during the post–World War II baby boom) and are now entering or passing through this stage of life.

The number of perimenopausal women in the United States has almost doubled in the past fifty years (see the figure below representing the U.S. Census Bureau statistics). And it is projected that the number of women in hormonal transition will remain high over the next fifty years.

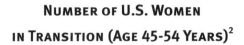

NUMBER OF U.S. WOMEN
IN TRANSITION (AGE 45-54 YEARS)[2]

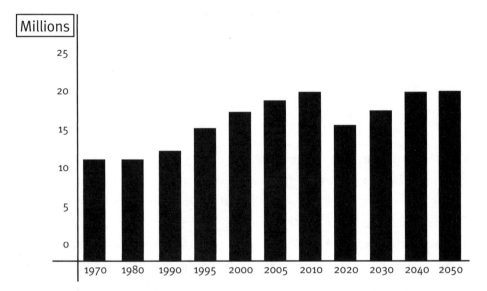

• Figures for 2000-2050 are projected.

   The life expectancy of women in the United States has increased while the average age of menopause has remained the same. Today, an American woman's average life expectancy is eighty years. The average age of menopause is 51.4 years. This means that American women—and women in similarly industrialized societies—will be spending more than one-third of their lives beyond menopause. There will be many more of us thinking about how to stay healthy as we age.

Chapter 5

The Effect of Estrogen on the Body's Organs

We have high levels of estrogen in our bodies during the young-adult years with beneficial effects on a number of organs. Estrogen exerts its influence on all the organs in our bodies and on all the other hormone glands. The ovaries, which produce estrogen, are hormone glands and function in sync with all of our other hormone glands, i.e., the pituitary, thyroid, thymus, and adrenal glands. Estrogen, like our other hormones, is protective and needed to maintain our health. It is widely dispersed throughout our bodies and estrogen levels affect our entire bodies. When estrogen levels fall, it changes the way we look and function. In my psychiatric practice, it's not unusual to have a woman referred for treatment for depression and insomnia without any recognition of these symptoms as being linked to hormonal changes. More commonly, these symptoms are attributed to a busy lifestyle and a mass of personal responsibilities. The point here is that midlife is marked by a constellation of changes which we can identify if we know what to look for.

The following is a partial list of symptoms that many women may experience but a few may not. Are you experiencing any of these signs and symptoms of estrogen depletion? Check the ones that apply to you.

_____ Irregular periods
_____ Hot flashes
_____ Mood swings
_____ Fragmented sleep
_____ Trouble concentrating
_____ Short-term memory loss
_____ Irritability
_____ Anxiety
_____ Depressed mood
_____ Reduced stamina
_____ Skin dryness
_____ Vaginal dryness
_____ Reduced sexual desire
_____ Breast sag
_____ Constipation
_____ Urinary tract infections
_____ Reduced muscle tone and weight gain
_____ Eye dryness
_____ Underactive thyroid, as shown by laboratory tests
_____ Gum infections and loose teeth
_____ Rise in cholesterol, as shown by laboratory tests
_____ Migraine headaches and new allergies
_____ Indigestion and bloating

Of interest is the fact that different symptoms are reported by different ethnic groups: for example, African-American women report hot flashes, night sweats, and forgetfulness as prominent symptoms; Caucasian women report sleeping problems and insomnia; Hispanic women report vaginal dryness, urine leakage, and pounding hearts as their most frequent symptoms; and

Asian-American women report their main symptom is memory loss (forgetfulness).

As you can see, we need our estrogen to keep us healthy, whether or not we're engaged in good health habits, and particularly in times of stress. The presence or absence of estrogen affects all the organs and organ systems.

Perimenopause, with its wildly fluctuating estrogen levels, is a transitional phase that has its own signs and symptoms. These are:

- Changes in the menstrual cycle: it can be heavier or lighter, longer or shorter, with bleeding between cycles
- Hot flashes and night sweats while still menstruating: studies report these in 25 to 33 percent of menstruating perimenopausal women; nonetheless, some physicians still mistakenly believe that hot flashes cannot occur in women who have sufficient estrogen to cause menstrual bleeding
- Problems with sexual functioning due to vaginal changes: vaginal dryness, pain and bleeding on intercourse, and loss of desire for sex
- Poor quality of sleep and/or insomnia: this is often due to night sweats interrupting the sleep pattern
- Forgetfulness, nervousness, and irritability: these are the symptoms that make many women fearful that they are losing mental capacity
- Intensification of any psychiatric symptoms that might be present: depression and anxiety symptoms will often reemerge even if the woman hasn't been experiencing these for some time

A woman can experience perimenopausal symptoms for eight to ten years prior to menopause. And, if the symptoms are multiple and severe enough, her quality of life can be seriously affected.

In addition, perimenopausal women with psychiatric disorders are prone to health problems in their postmenopause years. For example, the Johns Hopkins School of Public Health recently announced their findings from a study of clinically depressed women in hormonal transition. They found that these women had an increased risk of developing cancer in their first ten post-menopause years as compared to their nondepressed counterparts. Is there an as-yet-unexplained connection between chronic depression, declining estrogen levels, and cancer?

Chapter 6

Estrogen Withdrawal Symptoms

Sometime around the age of forty-five or fifty, we begin to experience the symptoms of lowered estrogen levels. The process of declining estrogen production can start much earlier for some and later for others.

There are three main forms of estrogen that occur naturally in women and are made in our ovaries:

- E1, or Estrone, is dominant in postmenopause and much less potent;
- E2, or Estradiol, which dominates during the reproductive years; and
- E3, or Estriol, which is dominant during pregnancy.

E1 and E2 can convert into each other. All three fluctuate wildly during perimenopause.

At midlife, the ovary doesn't stop producing estrogen. It goes through a shift, producing less potent estrogen with the aid of our fat cells and muscle tissue. The overall result is a continued production of estrogen by the ovaries, albeit at low maintenance levels. When a woman has both her ovaries removed, she loses this production capacity.

Some definitions:

- Perimenopause—the period of time prior to the cessation of menstruation during which many symptoms related to fluctuating hormones appear (average age of onset is forty-seven to fifty-one).
- Menopause—the last menstrual period (but we can't really identify this one for a year or so; average age is fifty-one).
- Postmenopause—the time following menopause when the symptoms of estrogen absence appear (there are three stages: early, age fifty-one to fifty-five; intermediate, age fifty-five to sixty-five; and late, over age sixty-five).

What are the biological markers that menopause is coming? The most common are:

- Decline in fertility with increased risk of miscarriages, premature labor, and stillbirths.
- Change in the pattern of the menstrual cycle: 90 percent of all women experience four to eight years of menstrual-cycle changes prior to menopause; irregular period is the most frequent symptom.
- Hot flashes/night sweats increase, affecting 85 percent of American women: for most women, they last three to five years, but for a few women, they can last ten to twenty years after menopause. They last longer and are more severe when menopause has been surgically induced. They are the second most frequently reported symptom.
- Insomnia is usually an inadequate amount or poor quality of sleep, which causes fatigue, concentration problems, and irritability.
- Urogenital changes: the vagina narrows and shortens, the lining thins and loses lubrication, and sexual stimulation decreases.

Within the first five postmenopause years, most women will have vaginal changes.

- Urinary problems: leakage of urine, increased frequency of urination (especially at night), and increased frequency of urinary-tract infections occurs in 30 percent of American women past the age of fifty.
- Changes in skin, eyes, hair, and teeth occur: we experience thinning and wrinkling of the skin and dry skin, dry eyes, sensitivity to light and poorer vision, thinning scalp hair, and gum disease and tooth loss (these are the early signs of osteoporosis).
- Short-term memory problems and difficulty concentrating begin: there are no good studies as to why, but the theory is that it is due to the impact of estrogen depletion on neuro-transmitters.
- Women with a history of psychiatric illness will have an exacerbation of that illness in menopause.
- There are other common symptoms experienced by midlife women, but these have not been proven to be caused by estrogen deficiency, but rather are believed to be caused by lifestyle and the process of aging aggravated by hormone deficiency. These are weight gain (experienced by 30–50 percent of American women), the joint pain of osteoarthritis, migraine headaches, and heart palpitations.

The majority of women have some perimenopause symptom and one in five of us have symptoms severe enough to disrupt our lives.

The best "test" for evaluating whether or not a woman is perimenopausal is the diagnostic interview. Many women are confused and upset by the complexity of the physical and emotional symptoms that can abruptly occur at midlife. I find that symptom questionnaires help explain the range of problems that can occur and help initiate the discussion of the impact of estrogen loss on our bodies as a whole. The Greene Climacteric Scale, for instance, is a brief and useful self-administered questionnaire that describes and rates the severity of each woman's symptoms in the following areas: psychological (anxiety and depression symptoms), vasomotor (sweating and hot flashes), somatic (other physical symptoms), and change in sexual interest. Sharing this important information about change of life symptoms is reassuring and often therapeutic.

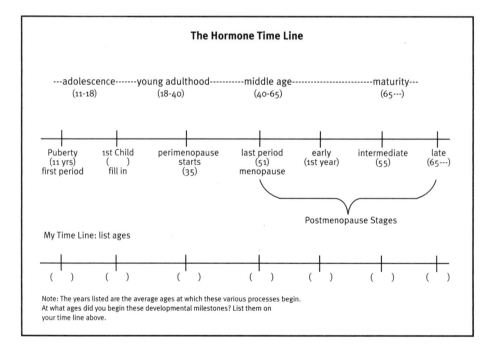

This is a daunting list of symptoms. Some women may experience a few or none of them. Estrogen is widely dispersed throughout the body and estrogen levels affect the entire body. When estrogen levels fall, the way we look and operate changes. These symptoms are often attributed to a busy lifestyle and a mass of personal responsibilities and not recognized as linked to hormonal changes. Again, the point here is that midlife is marked by a constellation of changes we can identify if we know what to look for.

Estrogen exerts beneficial actions in a number of tissues: it is a key hormone in the maintenance of the skeleton, of the brain, of cardiovascular integrity, in cancer prevention, in protection against tooth loss, and in protection from eye disease.

Midlife for both men and women is marked by high levels of stress (work, marital, and social). High levels of estrogen protect women from the physical damage that sustained periods of stress can cause. Stress coupled with hormonal changes will increase the intensity and severity of perimenopausal symptoms.

The following is a listing of the common symptoms that the majority of perimenopausal women will experience. One out of five women will have symptoms severe enough to adversely affect the quality of her relationships, work life, sexual functioning, and, eventually, her health. Unlike what we believed in the past, many perimenopausal symptoms can persist into our mature years.

Interestingly, medical research has learned more about the evolution of symptoms and physical change in women as we pass through this life phase because, in the last 150 years, our life expectancy has almost doubled. We no longer live into our early fifties but into our mid-eighties, yet the average age of menopause has not changed, remaining at fifty-one years. My point is this: women used to die at the end of their reproductive life span, but not any longer. And since we are living thirty to forty years past the onset of perimenopause, medical researchers have been able to evaluate women for these many symptoms and emerging health problems. It is only since the 1980s that knowledge of estrogen action has become available to an interested public.

The following are checklists of symptoms to help you identify where you might be along the menopausal transition.

PERIMENOPAUSAL SYMPTOMS
Check all that describe you.

Menstrual Period
_____ I am missing periods.
_____ My cycle is irregular.
_____ My periods are closer/further apart.
_____ My bleeding is heavier/lighter than previously.
_____ I am spotting between periods.
_____ My PMS symptoms are worse.

Hot Flashes
_____ Once a day or less, and they're manageable.
_____ More than once a day, and they occasionally interfere with my life.
_____ Every fifteen minutes, and they're driving me crazy.

Night Sweats, Insomnia
_____ Occasionally, I throw the covers off.
_____ Most nights, I wake up once drenched in sweat.
_____ I don't sleep as well as I used to.
_____ I can't function unless I get a full night's sleep.

Mood Swings

_____ I am more irritable than I used to be.

_____ I am fine one minute and then suddenly angry or depressed and then fine again.

_____ I'm nervous.

_____ I feel depressed.

_____ I'm crying a lot over little things.

_____ I'm exhausted.

Vaginal Dryness

_____ Intercourse is a little uncomfortable, my vagina is dry.

_____ I am uncomfortable during intercourse but fine otherwise.

_____ My vaginal area itches.

_____ I'm getting a lot of vaginal infections.

Other Symptoms

_____ I have lost my interest in sex and that devastates me.

_____ My thinking seems fuzzy.

_____ I can't concentrate.

_____ My memory is poor.

_____ I have headaches.

_____ I am gaining weight.

_____ My skin is dry and wrinkly.

_____ I have heart palpitations and shortness of breath.

_____ I feel dizzy.

_____ My joints ache.

MENOPAUSAL AND POSTMENOPAUSAL SYMPTOMS

Check all that describe you.

Early Stage (includes menopause and the first few
                postmenopause years)

__✓__ My period has completely stopped.

_____ I haven't had a period in twelve months.

__✓__ I have hot flashes and night sweats.

_____ I am unable to fall asleep or stay asleep as I used to.

_____ I am irritable and short-tempered.

__✓__ I am depressed.

Intermediate Stage (marked by physical changes)

_____ I can't even consider intercourse because of the pain/
       bleeding involved.

_____ I have cystitis.

_____ I urinate frequently.

_____ My urine leaks when I sneeze/cough/laugh/make love.

_____ I wear a pad to protect my underwear from urine spotting.

_____ My skin on my hands/face/neck (the areas where skin is
       exposed to the sun) is wrinkled.

__✓__ I've gained weight that I can't lose.

_____ I'm physically weaker.

__✓__ My eyesight has gotten worse.

__✓__ My hair is thinning/graying.

__✓__ My memory lapses are disturbing to me.

_____ I have gum disease and tooth loss.

The difference between these symptoms and those of peri-menopause is that these are persistent and more likely to be permanent.

Late Stage (diseases I have been diagnosed with)

_____ Coronary artery disease

_____ High blood pressure

_____ Osteopenia/Osteoporosis

_____ Thyroid disease

_____ Macular Degeneration of the eye *Eye problem*

_____ Diabetes, Type II

_____ Osteoarthritis

_____ Cancer (breast, uterine, ovarian, or colon)

_____ Alzheimer's disease *worry about*

_____ Hypercholesterolemia
(Elevated serum cholesterol/triglycerides)

Chapter 7

Postpartum Blues and PMS
The Other Significant Syndromes Caused by Hormone Dysfunction

There are two significant syndromes besides perimenopause/ menopause that are caused by hormone dysfunction, and up to 80 percent of women will experience either or both. These are Postpartum Blues and PMS.

Postpartum Blues

Postpartum Blues is believed to be due to the rapid decline of estrogen immediately after giving birth and for up to two weeks thereafter. It usually begins on the third or fourth postpartum day and ends spontaneously by the end of the second week.

On the third day home from the hospital after delivering our firstborn, my husband came home to find me in tears, moaning, "I'm a bad mother." He tried to be sympathetic, but basically told me to remember my understanding of medicine. We are all anxious to be good mothers, but my collapse into tears and self-deprecation had a biological base: my estrogen levels had plummeted, and I was feeling it.

Quiz

Did you have any of these symptoms after giving birth? Check
 those that apply:

_____ Depression

_____ Mood swings

_____ Anxiety

_____ Crying

_____ Sleep problems

_____ Poor concentration

CIRCLE YES OR NO

Did your symptoms interfere with taking care
   of your child?   Y   N
Were you ever treated for postpartum depression,
   a more severe form of the blues, which can last
   many months after delivery?   Y   N

If you answered "yes" to either of the above questions, it is likely
that depression will be one of your most debilitating perimenopausal symptoms.

Postpartum Depression

Most women (80 to 85 percent) will experience mood changes
after giving birth and they pass within a few days. Postpartum
depression, however, is persistent depression with symptoms that
occur after childbirth and last more than two weeks. One out of
eight postpartum women experience this form of depression. We
believe that those women most at risk for this form of depression
are those with:

- A prior history of depression;
- A family history of depression and/or bipolar disorder;
- Poor social support, i.e., marital discord;
- A childhood history of neglect or loss of a parent;
- Depressed mood during pregnancy;
- Stressful life events; or
- A history of PMS.

Premenstrual Syndrome (PMS)

PMS is the most common health problem experienced by women, and it starts in puberty. We don't know its cause, but we know that estrogen fluctuation is a major factor. PMS symptoms can be severe enough to impair our functioning, and they can persist until menopause.

Student Lauren Avera has written an interesting, unpublished paper on PMS. It is the source of the discussion that follows.

There are three main hormones whose effects manifest themselves during a woman's menstrual cycle (see chapter 3). These hormones affect mood, energy level, thought processes, sexual desires, eating behavior, and quality of sleep. They also induce various physical symptoms. Each hormone has a corresponding receptor area in the brain and can affect the production of neurotransmitters that regulate mood and behavior. These hormones also have an effect on other mood-altering substances called neuropeptides. Having improper levels of these hormones can increase the intensity of a woman's premenstrual symptoms.

PMS refers to an array of emotional, cognitive, physical, and behavioral symptoms that occur during the premenstrual phase of a woman's cycle. Researchers have identified about 150 symptoms that women experience during the menstrual cycle. They have isolated the most common, which produced a list of eighty-eight symptoms; and they put those symptoms into five categories: cognitive, emotional, physical, sexual, and behavioral.

The cognitive symptom grouping reflects the fact that PMS interferes, to one degree or another, with thinking, attentiveness, concentration, ability to plan ahead, and ability to reason in stressful situations.

The emotional grouping reflects the fact that PMS impacts emotional sensitivity: PMS heightens it. During the luteal phase of the menstrual cycle, a woman may experience noticeable emotional shifts, becoming irritable, then tense, then depressed, then something else.

The physical grouping reflects the fact that physical symptoms of varying intensity result from physiological changes that occur naturally during a woman's menstrual cycle.

The sexual grouping reflects the fact that there seems to be an increase in sexual desire, but often a decrease in sexual activity during the luteal phase.

The behavioral grouping reflects such things as the increases in eating and drinking and the cravings for sweet and salty foods that occur.

These symptoms differ in degree in terms of discomfort. There are generally three levels of discomfort. The first is termed "mild," which means that PMS symptoms are not interfering with ordinary daily activities. The second is termed "moderate," which means that PMS symptoms are interfering to a slight degree with ordinary daily activities. The third level of discomfort is termed "severe," which means that ordinary daily functioning is impaired.

It is the interaction among the pituitary and hypothalamus glands and the ovaries that governs the amount of hormones released into the bloodstream. This interaction is affected by a number of environmental factors such as stress, diet, socioeconomic status, emotional makeup, and physiological makeup.

One of the definitions of PMS is premenstrual stress. There are basically four categories of things that generate a stress reaction. These clusters of stressors require the body to perceive, process, and respond to changes.

The first category consists of situational stressors. This set includes sources of stress that are related to such things as work, home life, personal finances, relationships, stage of development, and extended family conditions.

The second category consists of psychological stressors. This category covers such phenomena as conflict within one's self or with others, difficult life decisions, personal illness or illness of loved ones, significant disappointments, falling in love, falling out of love, and perceived failures and successes.

The third category consists of physiological stressors. This category includes such things as temporary medical problems (such as allergic reactions), ongoing medical problems (such as diabetes), and changes in the level of hormones (thyroid, adrenal, or ovarian).

The fourth category consists of environmental stressors, such as workplace conditions, the temperature and noise level in your general environment, your personal safety, and time and performance pressures.

In general, stress adversely affects the neurotransmitters that in turn affect a woman's ovarian functioning, leading to lowered estrogen. This can make it more difficult for us to cope with stress.

If you are still menstruating and you suffer from PMS, complete the daily symptom checklist that follows. It is likely that the PMS symptoms you've experienced will persist throughout perimenopause, with the addition of a few more.

PMS AND PERIMENOPAUSE SYMPTOMS IN COMMON
Check all that apply to you.

PMS		Perimenopause
_____	Headaches	_____
_____	Fatigue	_____
_____	Heart palpitations	_____
_____	Anxiety	_____
_____	Depression	_____
_____	Anger	_____
___✓___	Moodiness	___✓___
___✓___	Irritability	___✓___
___✓___	Poor concentration	___✓___
_____	Insomnia	_____
_____	Decreased sex drive	_____

DAILY SYMPTOM CHECKLIST FOR PMS

Name _____

If you are still menstruating, start keeping this checklist on the first day of your menstrual period. Each evening, rate your symptoms according to the scale at right.

Make two copies of this checklist. Fill it out for two complete menstrual cycles.

Scale
0 = Symptom is absent
1 = Symptom is mild
2 = Symptom is moderate
3 = Symptom is severe but you are
    able to function
4 = Symptom is severe and you are
    unable to function

Note Date																													
Day of menstrual cycle	1	2	3	4	5	6	7	8	9	10	11	12	13	14	15	16	17	18	19	20	21	22	23	24	25	26	27	28	29
Note mensus with M																													

Symptoms   Ratings according to scale above

1. _____																													
2. _____																													
3. _____																													
4. _____																													
5. _____																													

Take a moment now and turn to your Menopause Action Plan at the back of the book. Begin to complete the Plan, based on what we've looked at here in part I.

Part II

The Individual is the Context

Chapter 8

Your Medical History

Even though menopause is a natural event, some women need treatment for short-term symptoms and/or prevention of long-term disease. Some women who have severe symptoms are embarrassed to seek help and feel they've failed to control their health problems. Some women will choose no outside help, perhaps because they have no symptoms or they view the symptoms as temporary, minor discomforts. And some women treat their symptoms with over-the-counter products that they believe are safe, despite not having adequate, unbiased information.

Midlife can be an especially difficult time for so many women. As each woman experiences some menopause-related symptoms, there are several relevant issues:

- What is her view of menopause and aging?
- What is she experiencing, and what is her medical history?
- What have her female relatives experienced?
- Does she have any long-term health risk factors for cardiovascular disease, osteoporosis, or cancer?
- Does she need to modify her lifestyle and make some changes, such as in diet and exercise, or the addition of vitamin and mineral supplements?

- Does she have any special counseling needs in areas such as smoking cessation, sexual functioning, substance abuse, or symptom relief?
- Are there psychological and social needs, such as family relationships, job satisfaction, or financial concerns?

Each woman is unique—unique in her biological and psychological response to menopause and aging, in her tolerance for various symptoms, in her risk profile for disease as she matures, and in her attitudes about treatment for her symptoms.

The major source of information about menopause comes from consumer magazines, probably because they are more available than medical professionals who are perceived as more authoritative.

Surveys show that women have deficits and misunderstandings in their knowledge about menopause and in their knowledge about the health risks in the years after menopause. Other surveys indicate that women are divided in their views about menopause: half see it as a medical condition requiring treatment and half view it as a natural transition that should be managed by natural means.

There is a real need to clear up the misconceptions concerning the vast array of physical and emotional changes that occur during midlife. And, since the change of life is inevitable, it's not optional for any of us. Education, assessment, and risk management are essential; treatment may or may not be necessary.

The Visit to Your Doctor

When you go to your doctor's office for the first time, you'll have medical history forms to fill out. Some of the diseases we are at risk for in later life are genetic. You'll need to know if any family members have had any of these problems:

FAMILY HISTORY

Please indicate whether immediate relatives (parents, siblings, grandparents, aunts/uncles, cousins, or children) currently have or died from any of the following:

CANCER:
_____ Breast
_____ Ovarian
_____ Uterine
_____ Colon
_____ Cervical
___✓__ Other

OTHER FAMILY HEALTH HISTORY:
___✓__ High blood pressure
___✓__ Heart attack
_____ Diabetes
_____ Osteoporosis
___✓__ Alzheimer's
___✓__ Mental illness

_____ Obesity
_____ Stroke
_____ Other
_____
_____
_____

Your personal history is also important, so let's review your health status, starting from just before puberty. Genetics can play a role here also, so find out if other family females have had similar problems.

Developmental Milestones Questionnaire

Instructions: in the Self column, check all that apply to you. In the Others column, enter M for mother, S for sister, A for aunt, and O for any other biologically related females.

PREPUBERTY AND PUBERTY	SELF	OTHERS
Stayed under normal weight	_____	_____
Menses had stopped	_____	_____
Went on eating binges	_____	_____
Purged self	_____	_____
Fasted	_____	_____
MENARCHE (STARTS WITH THE 1ST PERIOD)		
Irritability	_____	_____
Depressed mood	_____	_____

Tension and anxiety	_____	_____
Increased carbohydrate craving	_____	_____

CIRCLE YES OR NO

Did any of these start at ovulation and end during bleeding? Y   N
Were they severe enough to interfere with school,
    work, social activities, or relationships?   Y   N

YOUNG ADULTHOOD

Did/do you have any of the following medical problems?

	SELF	OTHERS
Hypoglycemia	_____	_____
Fibromyalgia	_____	_____
Chronic fatigue	_____	_____
Environmental allergies	_____	_____
Irritable bowel syndrome	_____	_____
Migraine headaches	_____	_____
Chronic pelvic pain	_____	_____
PMS	_____	_____

CHILDBEARING YEARS

Treated for anxiety or depression	_____	_____
Postpartum blues	_____	_____
Medical complications during pregnancy and/or delivery	_____	_____

OLDER ADULT

Overweight	_____	_____
Menopause began before the age of 45	_____	_____
Had or are undergoing steroid therapy	_____	_____
Fractures of the hip, spine, or wrist	_____	_____

Lost height	_____	_____
Urinary tract infections	_____	_____
Persistent joint pain	_____	_____
Hearing or memory loss	_____	_____

How each of us experiences the change of life and emerges through it is influenced by our past — our past health.

The following Midlife Health Assessment puts emphasis on family genetics that can put us at risk for future disease: menstrual cycle problems from puberty through adulthood because these can become intensified during perimenopause; and early signs of medical/psychiatric disorders that can emerge at menopause and continue into the postmenopause years.

The current status checklist describes the most common complaints of menopausal women in those domains that are of greatest concern to us as women — physical appearance, emotional well-being, sexual satisfaction, and close personal relationships.

MIDLIFE HEALTH ASSESSMENT
DEMOGRAPHICS

Date of Birth: _____

Ethnic Group: _____

Marital Status:

_____Never married	_____Divorced
_____Married	_____Widowed
_____Separated	

Education:

_____Grade school or less	_____Some high school
_____HS diploma or GED	_____Vocational/technical degree

_____Some college   _____College degree
_____Some graduate study   _____Graduate degree
Occupation:
_____Full-time work   _____Part-time work
_____Retired   _____Unemployed, looking
_____Unemployed,   for work
    not looking for work

FAMILY HISTORY OF DISEASE

Does anyone in your family have a history of the following:

Hypertension	_____No	_____Yes
Diabetes	_____No	_____Yes
Heart Disease	_____No	✓ Yes
Stroke	_____No	✓ Yes
Cancer		
Breast	_____No	_____Yes
Cervix	_____No	_____Yes
Colon	_____No	_____Yes
Endometrium	_____No	_____Yes
Lung	_____No	_____Yes
Ovary	_____No	_____Yes
Skin	_____No	_____Yes
Osteoporosis	_____No	✓ Yes
Alzheimer's disease	_____No	✓ Yes
Arthritis	_____No	_____Yes
Thyroid disease	_____No	_____Yes
Kidney disease	_____No	_____Yes
Blood clots	_____No	_____Yes

Bleeding disorders	_____No	_____Yes
Venereal disease	_____No	_____Yes
Clinical depression	_____No	__✓__Yes

DEVELOPMENTAL HISTORY (TEENAGE THROUGH MIDDLE AGE)

Teenage Years

How old were you when your period started? __14__

Around the time of your period, did you have any of these symptoms?

Irritability	_____No	_____Yes
Moodiness	_____No	__✓__Yes
Bloating	_____No	__✓__Yes
Breast tenderness	_____No	__✓__Yes
Binge eating	_____No	_____Yes
Purging	_____No	_____Yes
Fasting	_____No	_____Yes

How were your early periods characterized?

Regular	_____No	✓ _____Yes
Irregular	_____No	_____Yes
Light flow	_____No	_____Yes
Heavy flow	_____No	_____Yes
Cramps	_____No	__✓__Yes
No cramps	_____No	_____Yes
Short duration	_____No	__✓__Yes
Long duration	_____No	_____Yes

Habits:

Exercise	_____No	_____Yes
Smoking	_____No	_____Yes
Alcohol use	_____No	_____Yes

Other drug use   _____No   _____Yes
Sexually active   _____No   _____Yes
Hospitalizations and Surgeries:
    Date: _____   Reason: _____
    Date: _____   Reason: _____
    Date: _____   Reason: _____

Young Adult/Childbearing Years

Are you sexually active?   _____No   ✓Yes
Do you use birth control?   ✓No   _____Yes
Did/do you have any of the following medical problems?
    Hypoglycemia   _____No   _____Yes
    Fibromyalgia   _____No   _____Yes
    Chronic fatigue   _____No   _____Yes
    Environmental allergies _____No   _____Yes
    Irritable bowel syndrome _____No   _____Yes
    Migraine headache   _____No   _____Yes
    Chronic pelvic pain   _____No   __✓_Yes
    PMS   _____No   __✓_Yes
    Genital warts, Herpes,
       Syphilis (STDs)   _____No   _____Yes
    Depression/anxiety   _____No   ✓Yes
Pregnancies—How many?   _____
Abortions—How many?   _____
Miscarriages—How many?   _____
Number of children   _____
Medical complications during pregnancy or delivery? Describe:

_____

_____

Postpartum problems (depression? anxiety?) Describe:

_____

_____

Have there been any recent changes in your menstrual cycle?

Missed periods	_____No	_____Yes
Duration	_____No	_____Yes
Blood flow	_____No	_____Yes

Do you have any allergies?   _____No   _____Yes

Have you been treated for any medical/psychiatric disorders?

Date: _____	Reason:_____
Date: _____	Reason:_____
Date: _____	Reason:_____

Habits:

Exercise	_____No	_____Yes	_____Type
Smoking	_____No	_____Yes	
Caffeine	_____No	_____Yes	

How much coffee, tea, and soda do you drink daily?

_____

Alcohol   _____No   __✓__Yes

How much do you drink in a week?

_____*a glass per nights*_____

Other Drugs	Ever Used	Ever a Problem
Prescription	✓_____	_____
Narcotics	_____	_____
Cocaine	_____	_____
Crack	_____	_____
Heroin	_____	_____
Methadone	_____	_____
Marijuana	_____	_____

Tranquilizers   _____   _____
Sleeping pills   _____   _____
Amphetamines   _____   _____
LSD   _____   _____
PCP   _____   _____

Middle Age and Maturity

Have your periods stopped? _____No   _____Yes

If so, how old were you when you had your last period? 46

List all current medications:

Medication	Dosage	Reason
_____	_____	_____
_____	_____	_____
_____	_____	_____
_____	_____	_____

What is your current height? 5' 2"

What is your current weight? 115

Has there been a recent change in your height or weight?

                       ✓ No   _____Yes

Do you take vitamins/supplements/herbals?

                       _____No   ✓ Yes

Which exams do you have done yearly?

Pelvic   _____No   ✓ Yes
PAP   _____No   ✓ Yes
Mammogram   _____No   ✓ Yes
Eye   _____No   ✓ Yes
Blood pressure   _____No   ✓ Yes
Cholesterol   _____No   ✓ Yes

Current Status Checklist

Physical

Are you experiencing:

Changes in weight	_____No	__✓__Yes
Changes in energy	_____No	__✓__Yes
Changes in bowel habits	__✓__No	_____Yes
Changes in bladder functioning	__✓__No	_____Yes
Changes in sleep patterns	__✓__No	_____Yes
Frequent urinary infections	__✓__No	_____Yes
Decrease in muscle strength	_____No	__✓__Yes
Loss of muscle tone	_____No	__✓__Yes
Joint/muscle pain	_____No	__✓__Yes
Changes in eyesight	_____No	__✓__Yes
Skin dryness and wrinkling	_____No	__✓__Yes
Hair graying and thinning	_____No	__✓__Yes
Elevated cholesterol levels	_____No	__✓__Yes
Flushes of heat during the day	__✓__No	_____Yes
Profuse sweating at night	_____No	__✓__Yes

Emotional

Are you experiencing:

Worries concerning your health	_____No	__✓__Yes
Sudden appearance of physical complaints	_____No	__✓__Yes
Mood swings	_____No	__✓__Yes
Changes in memory and concentration	_____No	__✓__Yes
Depression/anxiety	_____No	__✓__Yes
Dissatisfaction with work/career	_____No	__✓__Yes

Dissatisfaction with your
    physical appearance   _____No   ✓_____Yes
Loss of confidence/feelings
    of inadequacy   _____No   _____Yes

Sexual

Are you experiencing:
    Decreased interest in sex   ✓_____No   _____Yes
    Decreased physical pleasure
        during intercourse   _____No   _____Yes
    Pain or dryness during intercourse   _____No   ✓_____Yes
    Inability to achieve orgasm   ✓_____No   _____Yes
    Decrease in sexual activity   ✓_____No   _____Yes
    Disappointment/anger toward
        your sexual partner   ✓_____No   _____Yes

Social (Relationships)

What is your current living arrangement?
    _____Alone   ✓_____Family/Spouse
    _____Significant Other   _____Caregiver
    _____Housemate(s)   _____Parent/Guardian
    _____Other

List the members of your household besides yourself:

Name	Age	Relationship
_____	____	_____
_____	____	_____
_____	____	_____
_____	____	_____
_____	____	_____

How long have you been with your current partner?

___✓___0–5 years _____5–10 years _____11+ years

Describe your satisfaction with your current relationship:

___✓___Extremely Satisfied

_____Fairly Satisfied

_____Fairly Dissatisfied

_____Not Satisfied

Are you involved in any community activities?

_____No ___✓___Yes

If yes, explain: _____

_____

Do you have any current, active religious affiliations?

___✓___No _____Yes

If yes, explain: _____

_____

Do you participate in any hobbies or leisure activities?

_____No ___✓___Yes

If yes, explain: _____

_____

Do you have close friends or family with whom you can discuss problems? _____No ___✓___Yes

If yes, explain: _____

_____

Chapter 9

Laboratory Tests and Screening Examinations

There is a persistent myth that since menopause is a natural, universal process, it must be healthy. This myth is very harmful. "Natural" does not mean that menopause has no serious health consequences. This may be so for some women, but not for all. Moreover, menopause is induced (by surgery, chemotherapy, irradiation, etc.) in a large number of women and therefore is not spontaneous or naturally occurring.

At menopause, our ovaries stop producing eggs and we have a dramatic decline in production of estrogen in our bodies. This results in an overall estrogen depletion. Estrogen affects every tissue in our bodies and there are receptor sites for estrogen on every organ in our bodies. It is essential to us. Specifically, we know that our own estrogen maintains our skeleton, improves cardiovascular functioning, gives us cancer protection (uterine and colon), helps with brain functioning, and protects us against tooth loss and eye disease. For some of us with high health risks and poor health habits, estrogen depletion can unmask early signs and symptoms of future disease.

The following are tests that you should have performed at the earliest appearance of change of life symptoms. Along with your physical exam, these will give you an evaluation of your physical functioning and state of health as you enter menopause. Following this list is an explanation of these tests and those internal organs that are being evaluated.

Lab Tests and Screening Exams

In addition to a physical exam (including a pelvic exam), the following tests should be performed. Write in your results.

LABORATORY TESTS

	Date	Results
Serum Glucose	_____	_____
Hemoglobin A1C	_____	_____
Cholesterol	_____	_____
HDL	_____	_____
LDL	_____	_____
Triglycerides	_____	_____
FSH	_____	_____
TSH	_____	_____
Mammography	_____	_____
Densitometry	_____	_____
Urinalysis	_____	_____
PAP	_____	_____
*Fecal Occult Blood	_____	_____
*Sigmoidoscopy	_____	_____
*STDs	_____	_____
GC	_____	_____
Chlamydia	_____	_____
BV/Yeast	_____	_____

HIV   _____   _____
*CRP   _____   _____
*If necessary, after discussion with your doctor

Your height will be measured on your first visit, and your weight and blood pressure every visit.

_____   Height
_____   Weight
_____   Blood pressure

Your weight should be such that you maintain a body mass index under 25 to avoid obesity (below 22 is ideal). Refer to chapter 35 in part V for a discussion of weight and body mass index, which takes into account both your *height* and your *weight*.

Your *blood pressure* is a measure of the pumping action of the heart. The top number is the *systolic* pressure (when the heart contracts) and the bottom number is the *diastolic* pressure (when the heart relaxes).

BLOOD PRESSURE GUIDELINES

Classification:	Systolic:	Diastolic:
Optimal	<120 mmHg	<80 mmHg
Prehypertensive	120–140 mmHg	80–90 mmHg
Hypertensive	>140 mmHg	>90 mmHg
*mmHg=mm of mercury		

A *serum glucose* test, or fasting blood sugar (FBS), is a blood test to detect diabetes. Normal FBS is below 126. A more sensitive blood test routinely administered to diabetics is the *Hemoglobin A1C*; a normal HgA1C is below 7 percent.

A *serum cholesterol* test is a blood test that measures the amount of fat circulating in your blood. *HDL* stands for high-density lipoprotein. HDL is called the "good" cholesterol because it helps remove fat from your bloodstream. *LDL* stands for low-density lipoprotein. LDL is called the "bad" cholesterol because it helps prevent fat from leaving your bloodstream, clogging your arteries. *Triglycerides* are other fats found in the bloodstream.

Optimal levels are:

Total cholesterol: under 200 mg/dl*

HDL: over 40 mg/dl

LDL: under 100 mg/dl

Triglycerides: under 150 mg/dl

*Mg/dl stands for milligrams of fat per deciliter of blood.

The *follicle-stimulating hormone (FSH)* test is used to diagnose menopause, although it is not a reliable test. If it is high, then ovarian functioning is believed to be low. It is not, however, reliable, because during perimenopause, false normal readings are common. Normal and postmenopause FSH levels in women are as follows:

Follicular Phase: 4.0–13.0 mcg/dl*

Ovulatory Phase: 5.0–22.0 mcg/dl

Luteal Phase: 2.0–13.0 mcg/dl

Postmenopause: 20.0–128.0 mcg/dl

*Mcg/dl stands for micrograms of FSH per deciliter of blood.

The test for *thyroid-stimulating hormone (TSH)* is a sensitive test for thyroid functioning. TSH is high if your thyroid is underactive (hypothyroidism) and low if your thyroid is overactive (hyperthyroidism). Complete thyroid testing is more extensive. Normal levels in women are:

> Thyroxine: 4.5–12.0 mcg/dl
> T3 Uptake: 20.0–47.0 percent
> TSH 0.38–4.70 mcIU/ml*
> Thyroxine, free: 0.7–1.9 mg/dl
> *McIU/ml stands for micro-International Units of TSH per milliliter of blood.

Mammography is an X-ray of the breasts to detect tumors too small to feel manually. The results will show any abnormal lumps or masses. It is effective but not infallible for early cancer detection. *Breast self-exam* is every woman's responsibility. The purpose is to detect lumps and changes in shape. The test is done by using your own hands; you will palpate your breasts in two positions; standing and lying down. Perform the test the same day every month. By performing the exam regularly, you'll get to know how your breasts are supposed to feel and be able to spot changes.

Densitometry is bone density measurement. It involves either an X-ray of the hip and spine or an ultrasound test of the heel or hand. It is used to detect bone loss as well as to measure the thickness and mineral content of bone (bone mineral density, or BMD). The ultrasound test gives a complete printout with results in two numbers: a Z-score comparing your bone mineral density to women in your age and ethnic group, and a T-score comparing your BMD to the average for Caucasian women between the ages of twenty-five and thirty-five, when bone density is at its peak. These scores are reported as standard deviations from the norm in each group; the norm is set at zero. You can be above or below the norm (plus or minus the mean).

Norms have not yet been developed for non-Caucasian women; until the studies are done, comparisons with Caucasian norms must suffice as approximations. The more important reading is the T-score.

The following interpretation is based on criteria set by the World Health Organization of the United Nations.

WHO Classification Criteria for T-Score Results

Classification	T-Score
Normal	Greater than –1.0
Low Bone Mass (Osteopenia)	Between –1.0 and –2.5
Osteoporosis	Less than or equal to –2.5
Severe or Established Osteoporosis	Less than or equal to –2.5 with the incidence of one or more low trauma fractures

Urinalysis is a test of fresh urine for the presence of blood cells and infectious organisms (as well as for sugar and protein content, as seen in diabetes). Urinary tract infections are common in women, and the midlife and older woman becomes increasingly susceptible to these infections.

A *PAP smear* is done to detect cancerous and precancerous cells on the cervix. The test is performed as part of a routine pelvic exam. The results will show where within three categories your cervical cells fall: negative, mild dysplasia, or positive for cancer. The purpose of a *pelvic exam* is to check on the health of your pelvic organs by manual examination. The test is done by your physician using his or her hands to examine your pelvic organs. The results will show whether fibroids, cysts, or infections are present.

At the discretion of your doctor, the following examinations can be performed.

The purpose of an *endometrial biopsy* is to determine the health of the lining of the uterus. Endometrial biopsies are usually performed in your doctor's office without an anesthetic by taking a small piece of tissue from the inner uterine wall. The tissue is examined for the presence of abnormal cells. Physicians recommend this test be scheduled prior to prescribing hormone replacement therapy (HRT).

The *fecal occult blood* test is a prescreening, an examination of your stool, prior to the ordering of a sigmoidoscopy or colonoscopy. *Sigmoidoscopy* and *colonoscopy* are screening tests for colon cancer and can be used to remove and examine polyps in the large intestine. These are performed after extensive cleansing of the bowel and done under anesthesia. Flexible tubing is inserted into the rectum and threaded up through the sigmoid and colon, an uncomfortable but painless procedure.

The test for *C-reactive protein (CRP)* is a relatively new blood test used to detect signs of heart disease. CRP is a protein produced by the liver to counter inflammation caused by damage to the walls of the arteries. It is a more sensitive test for heart disease and prediction of heart attack and stroke than is the test for cholesterol levels. Two consecutive readings are recommended.

Reading	Risk
Below 1.0 mg/l	Low risk
Between 1.0 and 3.0 mg/l	Moderate risk
Above 3.0 mg/l	High risk

Diagnosing Menopause with Laboratory Tests

The American College of Obstetrics and Gynecology issued a Practice Bulletin (2000) that stated that assaying follicle-stimulating hormone (FSH) levels in menopausal women may be a misleading indicator for determining menopause status. FSH levels are not a reliable predictor of where a woman is in this process because FSH levels can be low, normal, or high in perimenopausal women. FSH levels, however, can be indicative: a finding greater than 40 mcg/dl is suggestive that menopause is occurring.

Saliva hormone testing is now an available alternative to blood testing. It is a more accurate measure of the active hormones circulating in your body and available for use by your body. It is useful to check your hormone levels and to check on the effectiveness of your hormone replacement therapy. Like the blood test, it takes a week or two for the results to be available. It is expensive and not generally covered by insurance. You can ask your doctor about how to acquire a testing kit. I have seen them sold in product catalogues. One such kit is available at the following website: www.aswechange.com; the cost is $79.00.

Chapter 10

Recommended Tests and Screenings — By the Decade

Most of us get our medical information from radio, TV, and consumer magazines. When we're in the doctor's office, we might see a listing of screenings and medical tests we should have done. Some physicians will send us notices and reminders. Many of us are inconsistent, even haphazard, in having tests and screenings performed, no matter what our doctors recommend.

This chapter highlights the important tests to get during each decade of your life. From perimenopause through the post-menopause years, we will need to screen for bone mineral loss, heart and blood vessel disease, cancers, and eye disease because we are increasingly susceptible to diseases of our organs as we age. These diseases are the major causes of physical disability in the older woman. Screening provides early detection and help in preventing the organ damage that limits life and living.

Unless there are indications of disease.

When You're Thirty-Something

In your mid-thirties, your estrogen levels will begin to fluctuate, or go outside the levels your body is accustomed to in its normal cycle. You may begin to have hot flashes, or your periods may become heavy or irregular. You may begin to lose small amounts of bone mass. For some women, this is the onset of perimenopause.

- Get a physical every year that includes measurement of your blood pressure.
- Have your cholesterol levels tested at least every five years to look for warning signs of coronary artery disease.
- Have a PAP smear done to detect abnormalities. Have a pelvic exam annually to detect abnormalities of the uterus and ovaries.
- Examine your breasts monthly and get a mammogram, if you and your doctor feel it's necessary.
- If you are not committed to one sexual partner and he to you, get screened for Sexually Transmitted Diseases (STDs).

When You're Forty-Something

There is an increasing decline in estrogen levels and many women begin to have hot flashes, night sweats, irregular sleep, and irregular periods. The risk of heart disease increases, as does the loss of bone mineral density.

- Continue to have annual physical exams with blood-pressure readings.
- Have your cholesterol levels tested every three years.
- Get a pelvic exam and PAP smear annually.
- Have a mammogram done at least every two years.
- Continue monthly self-examination of your breasts.
- Begin colon cancer screening; have one done every three to five years.
- Screening for STDs is recommended.

When You're Fifty-Something

The average age of menopause today is fifty-one. Symptoms proliferate and include vaginal and urogenital problems. Bone loss is particularly rapid in the first seven years after menopause, and the risk of heart disease continues to increase.

- Continue your annual physicals with blood-pressure readings.
- Continue to have your cholesterol levels checked every three years, or get a CRP.
- Have a pelvic exam and PAP smear every year.
- Have a mammogram done every year.
- Get a bone mineral density (BMD) test done annually; the ultrasound screening is adequate.
- Continue to screen for colon cancer every three to five years.
- Have a sigmoidoscopy done every three to five years.

When You're Sixty-Something

There is an increase in vaginal dryness and related sexual problems. The incidence of osteoporosis, heart disease, and colon cancer increases.

- Continue your annual physicals with blood-pressure readings.
- Continue to have your cholesterol levels checked every three years, or get a CRP.
- Have a pelvic exam and PAP smear every year.
- Have a mammogram done every year.
- Continue your monthly self-examination of your breasts.
- Have a bone mineral density test done every three to five years.
- Begin having an eye exam and glaucoma screening every one to two years.

- Continue colon cancer screening every three to five years.
- Have a sigmoidoscopy every three to five years.

When You're Seventy-Something, or More

Eye conditions and cataracts become more common. This affects more women than men. The incidence of heart disease doubles, and your memory and cognitive functions may decline.

- Continue your annual physical with blood-pressure readings.
- Have your cholesterol levels checked at least every year, or get a CRP.
- Have a pelvic exam every one to three years.
- PAP smears are not needed if you are a woman older than sixty-five who historically has had normal results and are not at high risk for cervical cancer.
- Have a mammogram annually.
- Continue to examine your breasts monthly.
- Have a bone mineral density test done every three to five years.
- Continue eye examination and glaucoma screening every one to two years.
- Screen for colon cancer every one to two years.
- Have a sigmoidoscopy every three to five years.

Chapter 11

Early History Counts

Many medical and psychiatric disorders become reactivated or worsen during perimenopause. Moreover, they reinforce (read: aggravate) each other. The exception to this would be endometriosis, which actually improves with ovarian slowdown at menopause. Refer to "Your Medical History" in chapter 8. Have you had treatment for any medical/psychiatric problems in previous years? If so, list these conditions.

Adolescence: _____

Young Adulthood: _____

Childbearing Years: _____

Middle Age: _____

Over the years, I've had a lot of women referred to me who were experiencing midlife change and who were also diagnosed with a variety of psychiatric disorders. Let's look at a woman's life cycle from the point of view of our female reproductive milestones.

At puberty, whatever the age, girls become susceptible to eating disorders.

From adolescence through adulthood, we can experience depression, anxiety, premenstrual syndrome and its severe form, called *premenstrual dysphoric disorder (PMDD)*. For many women, PMS is experienced as an intense but brief time of depression and physical pain. About 80 percent of all women have mild or moderate symptoms, but only 5 percent have severe symptoms that actually interfere with or prevent daily functioning.

In the young adult years, there are conditions called *somatoform disorders*, so-called because of the predominance of physical symptoms. These are difficult to diagnose because physical examinations and laboratory studies and tests are usually negative. We have no effective treatment for these ailments. These conditions are hypoglycemia, fibromyalgia, chronic fatigue syndrome, environmental allergies, irritable bowel syndrome, atypical migraine headaches, and chronic pelvic pain.

During the childbearing years, women can also suffer from depression and anxiety. We are particularly susceptible to postpartum depression. Normally, up to 80 percent of postpartum women get "the maternity blues," which pass within two weeks.

The point is that, after puberty, all the major psychiatric disorders (mood disorders, anxiety disorders, somatoform disorders, and eating disorders) are common in women. In all these syndromes, the onset and severity of the symptoms are associated with times in the woman's hormonal cycle when the female hormones estrogen and progesterone are at low levels; that is, these conditions commonly occur in women with PMS, after childbirth, during the perimenopausal years, and in postmenopause. The wild fluctuation of our hormones during the perimenopause years can precipitate and intensify psychiatric symptoms. And, likewise, psychiatric disorders can trigger health problems in the maturing woman as hormone levels are rapidly depleted.

If a woman has a history of a psychiatric disorder, she will most likely experience an exacerbation of her symptoms at this time in her life. Conversely, the physical symptoms of perimenopause also have a domino effect; that is, untreated hot flashes and night sweats lead to sleeplessness and fatigue, resulting in irritability and an overall sense of loss of well-being, which, in turn, can precipitate symptoms of depression.

The number of symptoms that can occur is so large because estrogen is abundantly dispersed throughout our bodies and, during the menopausal years when our estrogen levels start to decline, all our organs are potentially affected.

Take a moment again and turn to your Menopause Action Plan at the back of the book. Complete that part of the Plan that reflects what we've examined here in part II. As you go on to part III, complete the assessments even for those diseases for which you are already being treated. Be sure to note the listing of factors that can be changed, because some of them might be helpful to your current treatment.

Part III

How's Your Health?

Chapter 12

Disease Risk Assessment

What makes up a disease risk assessment?

At midlife, many changes converge on us (and sometimes conspire against us): our bodies change, our families change, our social relationships change, and the sources of our emotional well-being change with them. Physically, our estrogen levels are declining; our ovaries are changing their function (explained in part I); we're losing estrogen's overall protective effect on our bodies; and the first early signs of future disease are emerging.

My own experience with perimenopause occurred over months with an accumulation of a variety of physical and emotional symptoms that became more intense as time went on. I thought my body was coming apart and, much worse, I thought I was developing medical illnesses over which I had no control. Thankfully, this crescendo of symptoms is mostly temporary; but these symptoms are signals to look more closely at our health status. This is the time of life when the accumulated years of bad habits and neglect begin to catch up with us. Some of our symptoms are not transient and are actually early signs of disease because they are tied to permanently diminished estrogen levels. Some of our symptoms are "silent" and are discovered as "accidental findings" on physical examination and screening tests: hence the importance of these evaluations at the first signs of perimenopause (see part II).

It's commonly agreed that women should get certain disease assessments at the change of life. Each assessment presented here is made up of those risk factors that can't be changed and those risk factors that can be changed. All significant factors are marked with a star. This is important because we can do a lot to influence our future health by making some simple lifestyle changes. Also of importance is the fact that many risk factors for these diseases overlap and, as we try to modify our risks for one disease, we can positively influence our risks for other diseases, as well. I've presented a rating system for use with the assessments, and I've also added a checklist of early signs and symptoms you should know about for many of these diseases.

The rating system has been devised to help you identify the importance and relevance to you of each assessment. The assessments don't rule in or rule out any physical illnesses. They do suggest further action you can take and point you in the direction of more evaluation. The ratings are *not* to be used as a substitute for a thorough medical evaluation and discussion with your doctor. They can help you focus on important medical issues and, used in combination with your medical history (see part II), you can focus your prevention strategies on current or future medical problems.

This is how the rating system works:

- *Insignificant Risk* means no action is necessary.
- *Low to Moderate Risk* means you have a combination of risks and possibly early symptoms of illness; you'll need to look closely at factors you can change and, if you are developing future problems, you should talk to your doctor.

- *Significant Risk* means you must act on this self-assessment by talking with your doctor and getting medical advice as soon as possible.

The following medical illnesses commonly occur in women, particularly as we age. Each is given its own chapter to make it easier to explain them, some in more detail than others. This is the list:

- Obesity
- Heart disease
- Hypertension and hypercholesterolemia
- Urogenital dysfunction
- Osteopenia and osteoporosis
- Thyroid disease
- Adult-onset diabetes
- Osteoarthritis
- Cancer (lung, breast, colon, uterine, cervical, and ovarian)
- Alzheimer's disease
- Depression and anxiety

There are risks for future health problems as we age. All women, young and old, need to know what these health problems are and what their risk factors for them are. Prevention can and should start early.

Years of neglect and putting off investigating subtle changes also start early. It is very easy to engage in the complexities of one's life and ignore or put off instituting good health habits. All of these medical conditions have specific risk factors, some of which are preventable and some of which aren't. It is important for women to find out what their individual risk factors are and to find out early enough in their lives so that they can take them into account as they plan for their future.

Even though these health problems express themselves in later life (in the fifties and beyond), the stage is set for the onset of these diseases much earlier in a woman's life. Knowledge about individual risks and education about prevention should start in the younger years. During the approximately fifteen years of perimenopause, a woman has a good opportunity to avert the adverse changes these conditions can wreak on her body in later life.

We are all aging, but the standards of normal aging have been revised. It is no longer the norm to accept the traditional concept of aging as gradually diminishing function (fading eyesight and hearing, impaired mental functioning, decreased strength and stamina). The new scenario of life after menopause is one of health and vigor. This book is aimed at just that. An evaluation of your quality of life and assessments of your current health and risks for future disease are the starting points.

In our thirties, we often take our quality of life for granted, but quality of life is a very real issue for women as we navigate the menopause transition. The quality of life we seek really means a sense of well-being in a variety of domains. As the first physical signs of menopause occur, many women are also experiencing change in other aspects of their lives. How well we navigate menopause and endure the physical symptoms of change of life has a lot to do with a sense of well-being in our overall health, our occupation, our emotional life, our sexual life, and in the quality of our relationships.

The Utian Quality of Life Scale was developed by researchers and perimenopausal women together. It is valid, reliable, and practical to use. This is a good assessment to take at any time in your life even though it was developed for use through and beyond menopause.

Here's how you use it.

Circle the number (1–5) that best describes you after each statement. Selection of the number 1 means the statement is not true of you; selection of the number 3 means the statement is moderately true of you; selection of the number 5 means the statement is very true of you. Total your scores within each factor (domain). Then, total your factor (domain) scores for an overall QOL score.

The factor total scores and overall scores have been computed five times to demonstrate how various factor total scores and overall scores are obtained.

THE UTIAN QUALITY OF LIFE SCALE

Factor 1. Occupational Quality of Life

I feel challenged in my work.	1	2	3	4	5
I believe my work benefits society.	1	2	3	4	5
I have gotten a lot of personal recognition at my job.	1	2	3	4	5
I am proud of my occupational accomplishments.	1	2	3	4	5
I consider my life stimulating.	1	2	3	4	5
I continue to set new personal goals for myself.	1	2	3	4	5
I continue to set new professional goals for myself.	1	2	3	4	5

Factor 2. Health Quality of Life

I am unhappy with my appearance.	1	2	3	4	5
My diet is not nutritionally sound.	1	2	3	4	5

I feel in control of my eating behavior.	1	2	3	4	5
Routinely, I engage in active exercise three or more times each week.	1	2	3	4	5
I believe I have no control over my physical health.	1	2	3	4	5
I feel physically well.	1	2	3	4	5
I feel physically fit.	1	2	3	4	5

Factor 3. Emotional Quality of Life

I am able to control things in my life that are important to me.	1	2	3	4	5
My mood is generally depressed.	1	2	3	4	5
I frequently experience anxiety.	1	2	3	4	5
Most things that happen to me are out of my control.	1	2	3	4	5
I expect that good things will happen in my life.	1	2	3	4	5

Factor 4. Sexual Quality of Life

I currently experience physical discomfort or pain during sexual activity.	1	2	3	4	5
I am not content with my sexual life.	1	2	3	4	5
I am content with my romantic life.	1	2	3	4	5
I am content with the frequency of my sexual interactions with a partner.	1	2	3	4	5

Totals

	Low		Moderate		High
Occupational QOL	7	14	21	28	35
Health QOL	7	14	21	28	35
Emotional QOL	6	12	18	24	30
Sexual QOL	3	6	9	12	15
Total QOL	23	46	69	92	115

There are many medical consequences of estrogen loss for women. The following is a brief discussion.

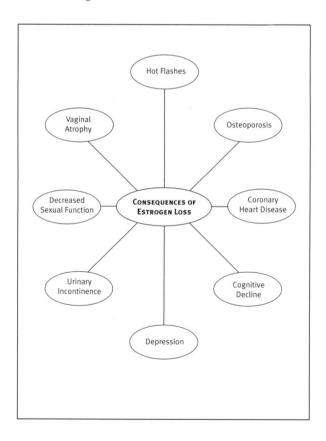

The major health concern for postmenopausal women is actually cardiovascular disease. While the cardiovascular death rates for men have decreased, they have increased for women.

Heart disease, coronary artery disease, and stroke are all rare in young women, but are the most frequent causes of death in women over age fifty. Most women, however, still believe that their major health concern is cancer. More women will eventually die of heart disease than of all the cancers combined. In fact, after the age of fifty, there is a sharp increase in occurrence of heart disease; one in two women will be affected.

LEADING CAUSES OF FEMALE DEATH
UNITED STATES, 2000

Cause of Death	Percent*
1. HEART DISEASE	29.9
2. CANCER	21.8
3. STROKE	8.4
4. CHRONIC LOWER RESPIRATORY DISEASES	5.1
5. DIABETES	3.1
6. INFLUENZA AND PNEUMONIA	3.0
7. ALZHEIMER'S DISEASE	2.9
8. UNINTENTIONAL INJURIES	2.8
9. KIDNEY DISEASE	1.6
10. SEPTICEMIA	1.4

*Percent of total deaths due to the cause indicated.

Table reproduced from ww.cdc.gov/od/spotlight/nwhw/lcod.htm.

The signs and symptoms of heart attacks (and of heart disease) in women are as follows:

- A tightness, squeezing, or pressure felt in the chest, upper abdomen, neck, throat, or jaw; may radiate down your left arm and cause a sensation of numbness or tingling
- Nausea or feelings of indigestion, including heartburn, sickness in the stomach, or general uneasiness
- Breathing difficulties without exertion
- Fatigue or an overall feeling of weakness and lack of energy

The genitourinary changes after menopause are caused by genitourinary atrophy, which in turn affects urinary and sexual functioning. It is a condition characterized by changes in the vagina and skin outside the vaginal opening, including vaginal dryness and shrinkage. In postmenopausal women, it is caused by loss of the estrogen previously produced by the ovaries. It is usually treated with estrogen replacement therapy. Externally applied creams have proven to produce good symptom control. All menopausal women will experience genitourinary atrophy and most will have urinary or sexual dysfunction. In my psychiatric practice, this is the least discussed consequence of change of life. The most common vaginal symptoms are burning, itching, pain, and decreased vaginal lubrication and elasticity. The most common urinary tract symptoms are urine leakage (incontinence) and frequent urination, especially at night.

Bone density in women also changes with age: it peaks in our twenties and starts to decline in our forties with rapid bone loss in our fifties. There is typically a 20 percent loss from the peak density by the age of sixty. Our bone density in our mature years is determined by how much bone was accumulated in our youth and the amount of bone loss during our middle years (see graph below). Bone loss in women who have undergone surgically induced menopause (from hysterectomies and oophorectomies) is an under-recognized and significant risk for osteoporosis.

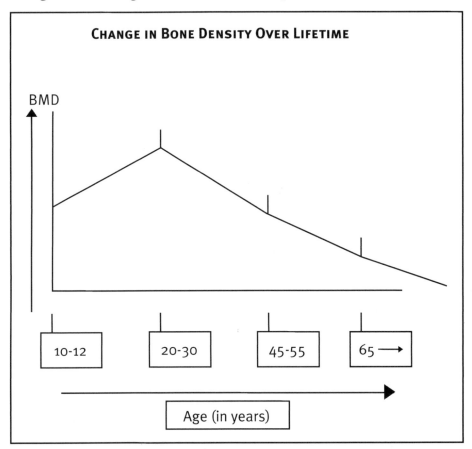

Cognitive decline, or slow and progressive loss of mental functioning, is not one of the leading disease risks faced by post-menopausal women. However, it is much more prevalent in women than in men and is a leading cause of institutionalization of women after the age of seventy. You may wish to screen yourself or someone you know.

Mild cognitive impairments can be detected early. Simple testing can reveal it. For example, counting backwards from 100 by 7s; spelling the word "world" backwards; or naming as many animals as you can in sixty seconds (eighteen or more is excellent; fewer than twelve is poor, as is naming something other than an animal); engaging another in conversation by asking: How are you? What do you like to do? and What did you do yesterday? (The inability to answer these questions implies cognitive impairment.) The Draw-a-Clock test asks that you draw a clock; those with cognitive impairment struggle to position the numbers around the clock face. Those with cognitive impairment asked to place the clock hands so as to indicate a specific time (for example, 9:25) will often misplace the hands on the clock.

Unlike cognitive impairments, forgetfulness is a normal part of aging. For a good explanation of memory and forgetfulness, refer to the following Harvard Health Publication: *Improving Memory: Understanding and Preventing Age-Related Memory Loss* (2000).

Depression is one of the conditions for which postmenopausal women are statistically at risk. I specialize in treating mood disorders, and I use several screening tools to assess depression symptoms in my patients. The one at the end of the chapter is self-administered. Scoring is done by adding all the points together. A score greater than one hundred is significant and suggests you should consider talking to a therapist.

DEPRESSION SCALE, PATIENT VERSION

Please rate how you have been feeling   Date _____
during the past week, including today.   Your Name _____

Key: 0-Absent 1-Mild 2-Moderate 3-Marked 4-Severe

	0	1	2	3	4
1. Depressed, sad	0	1	2	3	4
2. I am so depressed that not even good news would cheer me up	0	1	2	3	4
3. Angry, irritable, hostile	0	1	2	3	4
4. Decreased self-esteem or self-confidence, low thoughts about myself	0	1	2	3	4
5. Guilt feelings, feeling like a burden to family and society	0	1	2	3	4
6. Hopelessness, things will not get better	0	1	2	3	4
7. Helplessness, I can't change things	0	1	2	3	4
8. Trouble falling asleep	0	1	2	3	4
9. Waking up in the middle of the night	0	1	2	3	4
10. Waking up in the morning 1-2 hours before I need to	0	1	2	3	4
11. Sleeping more than usual	0	1	2	3	4
12. Drowsy during the day	0	1	2	3	4
13. Fatigue, low energy, hard to get going	0	1	2	3	4
14. Decreased appetite	0	1	2	3	4
15. Increased appetite	0	1	2	3	4
16. Decreased weight	0	1	2	3	4
17. Increased weight	0	1	2	3	4
18. Decreased sexual interest	0	1	2	3	4
19. Increased sexual interest	0	1	2	3	4
20. Decreased interest in usual activities	0	1	2	3	4
21. Decreased involvement in usual activities - withdrawn	0	1	2	3	4
22. Decreased pleasure or less enjoyment of usual activities	0	1	2	3	4
23. Decreased memory	0	1	2	3	4
24. Decreased concentration	0	1	2	3	4
25. Indecisiveness - unable to make decisions	0	1	2	3	4

26. I move slower; sit in one place for long periods	0	1	2	3	4
27. So restless I can't sit still or relax	0	1	2	3	4
28. Thoughts slowed down	0	1	2	3	4
29. Racing thoughts	0	1	2	3	4
30. Mood worse in morning	0	1	2	3	4
31. Mood worse in evening	0	1	2	3	4
32. My mood changes very rapidly	0	1	2	3	4
33. Thoughts of suicide, wishing I were dead, not caring if I live	0	1	2	3	4
34. Intent to kill myself	0	1	2	3	4
35. Wanting to hurt or punish myself (not suicide)	0	1	2	3	4
36. Anxious, nervous, worried	0	1	2	3	4
37. Physical anxiety symptoms like my heart beating oddly, short of breath, tremors, butterflies in my stomach, frequent urination, sweating, muscle tension, numbness in my hands or feet	0	1	2	3	4
38. So afraid of certain things or situations that I avoid them	0	1	2	3	4
39. Sudden, severe feelings that something is going to happen, like I will die, go crazy, or pass out	0	1	2	3	4
40. Hearing voices or seeing things that are not there	0	1	2	3	4
41. Believing things that others do not believe	0	1	2	3	4
42. Feeling suspicious of others, that others want to hurt me or are against me	0	1	2	3	4
43. Unpleasant, unrealistic thoughts go over and over in my mind and I can't stop them	0	1	2	3	4
44. Feeling compelled to do senseless things over and over	0	1	2	3	4
45. Feeling I am some other person or am outside my body	0	1	2	3	4
46. Feeling things are not real, like in a fog or dream world	0	1	2	3	4
47. Worried about my physical health	0	1	2	3	4
48. Feeling rejected by others	0	1	2	3	4
49. Unable to control my impulses	0	1	2	3	4
50. Drinking alcohol or using recreational drugs	0	1	2	3	4

Reproduced courtesy of the Feighner Research Institute.

The Women's Health Initiative is studying the impact of estrogen loss on the eyes. Age-related macular degeneration (AMD), though not one of the leading disease risks faced by postmenopausal women, is the leading cause of blindness in the United States among men and women alike. The common eye symptoms associated with menopause are deterioration in vision and dryness. Other age-related conditions are cataracts and glaucoma. The findings of the WHI are expected to greatly expand our knowledge of the impact of estrogen loss on such diseases of the eye.

Chapter 13

Obesity

Obesity is defined as a body mass index (see part 5, chapter 35) equal to or greater than 30.

Most women gain weight during the perimenopause and early menopause years due to increased fat storage as a result of metabolic change at this age. Have you noticed the new areas of fat pads on your back, arms, waist, and hips?

Two-thirds of women aged fifty and older are overweight (BMI of 25 or more) and half of these are obese. Weight gain is pervasive and occurs during perimenopause exclusively in Western societies. This is due to our four-decade-long habit of overeating, coupled with the metabolic change that occurs at this age. It is a slow, insidious process, and it shouldn't be ignored. A BMI at 30 or greater maintained for three years can cause increased blood pressure, increased blood sugar, and lipid abnormalities; after ten years, coronary artery disease will develop. Most importantly, obesity is either a major causative factor or a significant symptom in each of the diseases listed, except for Alzheimer's disease.

OBESITY RISK ASSESSMENT
Non-Changeable Risk Factors
Check each factor that describes you.

_____You have polycystic ovarian syndrome.*

_____You have hypothyroidism.*

_____ You are age fifty or older.

_____ You have a family history of obesity.

_____ Your body fat is distributed primarily throughout your abdomen, hips, and buttocks.

Risk Rating
No checks: Insignificant risk, no action needed at this time

One or more checks: Low to moderate risk, discuss with doctor at next exam

*Significant risk, discuss with doctor immediately

OBESITY RISK ASSESSMENT
Changeable Risk Factors
Check each factor that describes you.

_____ You are physically inactive (a couch potato).*

_____ You overeat and eat oversized portions.*

_____ You have more than two alcoholic drinks a day.*

_____ You are taking medications such as: antidepressants, anti-histamines, beta-blockers, analgesics, chemotherapy drugs, sulfonylureas for diabetes, steroids, anti-epileptic drugs, or contraceptives.*

_____ You frequently diet and skip meals.

_____ You eat few dairy products (and may have a calcium deficiency).

_____ You eat carbohydrate-rich foods (starches and sweets) daily.

_____ Body fat has accumulated in your abdomen (you have an apple-shaped body) or in your hips (you have a pear-shaped body).

_____ You were overweight prior to menopause.

_____ You smoke.

Risk Rating

Fewer than three checks: Insignificant risk, no action needed at this time

Three or more checks: Low to moderate risk, discuss with doctor at next exam

*Significant risk, discuss with doctor immediately

EARLY SIGNS OF OBESITY

Check each factor that describes you.

_____ Your appetite has been increasing.*

_____ You have been gaining more than five pounds of weight each year.*

_____ Your physical activity has been decreasing.*

_____ You drink more soda than water.

_____ You have increased your snacking on "junk foods," (potato chips, cookies, candy, cake).

_____ You eat fast food.

_____ You are unable to lose weight by dieting.

Risk Rating

Less than three checks: Insignificant risk, no action needed at this time

Three or more checks: Low to moderate risk, discuss with doctor at next exam

*Significant risk, discuss with doctor immediately

Chapter 14

Heart Disease, Hypertension, and Cholesterol

First, some definitions.

CVD stands for cardiovascular disease and refers to those processes that damage the heart and blood vessels. CHD stands for coronary heart disease and is often used interchangeably with CAD, which stands for coronary artery disease. CHD and CAD refer to diffuse buildup of plaque in your arteries, causing inflammation, hardening of the arteries, and atherosclerosis. CVD, CHD, and CAD stand for vascular and heart disease, and they mean their proud owner has a future risk of angina, TIAs (transient ischemic attacks), myocardial infarction (MI, or heart attack), and stroke. If we don't die from these conditions, we will probably need blood-thinners, bypass surgery, or other high-tech medical procedures to save our lives.

Our ovarian estrogen has many important functions (refer to part I): it acts as an antioxidant and prevents the buildup of "bad cholesterol" (LDL) in the blood vessel walls; it keeps the "good cholesterol" (HDL) at high levels, which delays hardening of the arteries; and it strengthens the heart muscle — all of which help to delay the onset of cardiovascular disease. Because women at menopause have a significant reduction in estrogen levels, our risk of heart disease increases dramatically in the postmenopause years (two to three times more so than in men). Therefore, one woman in nine between the ages of forty-five and sixty-four is estimated to have CHD; after age sixty-five this increases to one in three women. The loss of ovarian function for any reason (e.g., surgery, chemotherapy, early menopause) will also increase our risk for heart disease. Thus, for women between age fifty and seventy-five, heart disease is the leading cause of death (five times more common than death from breast cancer). Stroke is the second-leading cause of death and the most common cause of long-term disability in women in this age group.

The hardening of our arteries is a normal part of aging (but high cholesterol levels are not), and it leads to high blood pressure, which is the most common chronic condition in the United States. The combination of hardening arteries, fatty buildup in the walls of the arteries, and inflammation of the artery walls causes heart attack and stroke. Hypertension develops insidiously over time. It is estimated that one in four adults have it, and most of these people are women. If you're over the age of fifty-five, your risk of developing high blood pressure is 90 percent. And it's usually discovered by accident at routine physical exams. Hypertension doesn't make you feel sick the way high blood sugar does. Therefore, it's called the "silent disease." But if left untreated, it can kill you suddenly, without warning.

More than 50 percent of women over the age of fifty-five have high cholesterol. Even if you are not overweight, you can still have abnormal cholesterol levels. HDL ("good cholesterol") levels tend to decrease in the postmenopause years. Therefore, low levels of HDL are a much better indicator of heart disease risk in women than high levels of LDL (which is a more useful indicator of risk in men). Our bodies can make all the cholesterol we need. Some of us have a genetic predisposition to overproduction of cholesterol, but most of us get high levels of cholesterol from diets high in starches and fats.

Current Concepts

Hypertension is a chronic condition that affects one in four American adults, most of them women. The National Heart, Lung, and Blood Institute has issued new guidelines (2003) that will affect millions of us. A blood pressure reading of 120 systolic over 80 diastolic used to be considered ideal; now, it is considered borderline hypertensive. In other words, this blood pressure level isn't low enough. Most people don't know that they have high blood pressure until they develop symptoms. This usually means some damage has already occurred to the heart, kidneys, eyes, and brain.

The following are the new guidelines for *detecting* hypertension:

Pressure	Normal	Pre-Hypertensive	Stage I	Stage II
Systolic	‹120	120–139	140–159	›160
Diastolic	‹80	80–89	90–99	›100

Recommended **treatment** regimens are:

Healthy	None	Lose weight Exercise Avoid Salt and Alcohol	Diuretics	Diuretic + Another Drug
With Disease	None	Medically Treat	Multiple Meds	Multiple Meds

The relevant diseases here are heart disease, diabetes, and kidney disease.

Have your blood pressure checked at least twice yearly. Two or more consecutive high readings may indicate a problem is developing.

HEART DISEASE RISK ASSESSMENT

Non-Changeable Risk Factors

Check each factor that describes you.

_____ You have had a hysterectomy, chemotherapy, or early menopause.*

_____ You have had a heart attack.*

_____ You have had a stroke or transient ischemic attack (TIA).*

_____ You have diabetes.*

_____ You have kidney disease.*

_____ You are age fifty or older.

_____ You have a family history of heart disease.

_____ You have a family history of stroke.

_____ You have sickle cell anemia.

Risk Rating

No checks: Insignificant risk, no action needed at this time

One or more checks: Low to moderate risk, discuss with doctor
at next exam

*Significant risk, discuss with doctor immediately

HEART DISEASE RISK ASSESSMENT

Changeable Risk Factors

Check each factor that describes you.

_____ You have high blood pressure, as shown by two or more consecutive elevated readings.*

_____ You have high cholesterol, as shown by laboratory testing.*
_____ You are twenty pounds or more overweight.*
_____ You are physically inactive.
_____ You drink more than two alcoholic beverages a day.
_____ You smoke.
_____ You suffer from depression.

Risk Rating

Less than two checks: Insignificant risk, no action needed at this time
Two or more checks: Low to moderate risk, discuss with doctor
at next exam
*Significant risk, discuss with doctor immediately

EARLY SIGNS OF HEART DISEASE

Check each factor that describes you.

_____ You have had an angina attack (pain in abdomen, back, neck, jaw, or throat).*
_____ You suffer from nausea, indigestion, and heartburn.*
_____ You experience shortness of breath without exertion.*
_____ You have a lack of energy and feel weak and fatigued.*

*These all represent significant risk. Please note that they differ from typical signs such as chest pain radiating down the arm, often seen in men.

HYPERTENSION RISK ASSESSMENT

Non-Changeable Risk Factors
Check each factor that describes you.

_____ You are age sixty-five or older.*
_____ You have a family history of hypertension.*
_____ You have a family history of high cholesterol.*

_____ You have diabetes.*

_____ You have asthma.

_____ You are African-American.

Risk Rating

No checks: Insignificant risk, no action needed at this time

One check: Low to moderate risk, discuss with doctor at next exam

*Significant risk, discuss with doctor immediately

HYPERTENSION RISK ASSESSMENT

Changeable Risk Factors

Check each factor that describes you.

_____ You have a diet high in salt and fat (low in fruits and vegetables).*

_____ Your diet is poor in calcium-rich foods (see part V, chapter 32).*

_____ You are physically inactive.*

_____ You smoke.*

_____ You are obese.*

_____ You drink more than four cups of caffeinated coffee or other caffeinated beverages each day.

_____ You drink more than two alcoholic beverages a day.

_____ You use oral contraceptives.

_____ You are under chronic stress.

Risk Rating

Less than three checks: Insignificant risk, no action needed at this time

Three or more checks: Low to moderate risk, discuss with doctor at next exam

*Significant risk, discuss with doctor immediately

Early Signs of Hypertension

There are no early signs of hypertension. It is usually "discovered" by blood pressure readings taken on physical examination. Two or more consecutive high readings are needed to confirm the diagnosis.

HYPERCHOLESTEROLEMIA RISK ASSESSMENT

Non-Changeable Risk Factors

Check each factor that describes you.

_____ You have reached menopause, naturally or induced.*

_____ You are at least two years postmenopause.*

_____ You have diabetes.*

_____ You have a family history of high cholesterol.*

*Significant risk, discuss with doctor immediately

HYPERCHOLESTEROLEMIA RISK ASSESSMENT

Changeable Risk Factors

Check each factor that describes you.

_____ You are obese.*

*Significant risk, discuss with doctor immediately

EARLY SIGNS OF HYPERCHOLESTEROLEMIA

There are no early signs of high cholesterol. It is usually "discovered" by blood tests of cholesterol levels ordered by your doctor as part of a physical examination.

Chapter 15

Urogenital Dysfunction

Seventy-five percent of postmenopausal women have experienced changes in the functioning of their urinary tract as well as changes in their sexual functioning, but only one out of ten women will seek medical attention. And three out of ten will have permanent problems. Estrogen deficiency in the postmenopausal years causes the following impairments in the genitourinary tract:

- Vaginal dryness, shrinkage, and proneness to infection (known as atrophy)
- Urinary tract loss of elasticity and tissue shrinkage with proneness to infection and incontinence (known as atrophy)
- Sexual dysfunction due to pain and bleeding on intercourse, with loss of libido

Men and women are embarrassed and ashamed to admit to having any problems with sexual functioning. But women differ from men in how we handle these problems when they arise.

Rarely does a woman initiate discussion of these problems. In my psychiatric practice, I am usually the one to bring out these issues during the interview. Women tend to assume that sexual dysfunction is an emotional impairment; men tend to assume that it's a physical problem.

Women usually attribute problems with sex to stress in their lives; men usually attribute these problems to their sexual partners (they blame the partner).

Even though sexual dysfunction is one of the most common symptoms of menopause, women rarely recognize it as such, whereas in men, sexual dysfunction is often a sign of medical illness, for example, diabetes or prostate disease.

Women rarely seek medical help for sexual dysfunction unless the symptoms significantly interfere with their sexual functioning, whereas men tend to consult doctors earlier about signs of difficulties.

The key to treating these symptoms is early recognition of the problem. Please note that under the listing of vaginal signs, all are starred, meaning that if you are experiencing any of these symptoms, you will need to discuss the matter with your doctor.

UROGENITAL DYSFUNCTION RISK ASSESSMENT

Non-Changeable Risk Factors

Check each factor that describes you.

_____ You have been postmenopausal for at least one year, or are older than fifty.*

_____ You have had an injury to your pelvic nerves due to surgery, chemotherapy, or irradiation.*

_____ You have Crohn's inflammatory bowel disease.*

_____ You have allergies to soaps and deodorants.

_____ You suffer from skin disorders (for example, eczema).

_____ A sexually transmitted disease (for example, HIV) is present in your body.

Risk Rating

Less than two checks: Insignificant risk, no action needed at this time

Two or more checks: Low to moderate risk, discuss with doctor at next exam

*Significant risk, discuss with doctor immediately

UROGENITAL DYSFUNCTION RISK ASSESSMENT

Changeable Risk Factors

Check each factor that describes you.

_____ You are taking blood pressure medication, antidepressants, or antibiotics regularly.*

_____ You are obese.*

_____ You do not have a sexual partner.*

_____ You have low androgen levels as measured by blood testing for hormone levels.*

_____ You have seen the emergence of health problems, for example, high blood pressure, diabetes, and thyroid dysfunction.*

_____ You suffer from sleep disturbances.

_____ You suffer from depression.

_____ You smoke.

Risk Rating

Less than two checks: Insignificant risk, no action needed at this time

Two or more checks: Low to moderate risk, discuss with doctor at next exam

*Significant risk, discuss with doctor immediately

EARLY SIGNS OF UROGENITAL DYSFUNCTION
Vaginal Signs

Check each factor that describes you.

_____ You suffer from pain during intercourse.*

_____ You have decreased vaginal lubrication.*

_____ You have itching or burning in the vaginal area.*

_____ You have vaginal discharge regularly.*

_____ You have vaginal infections and urinary tract infections.*

_____ You suffer vaginal pain or dryness in the absence of sexual activity.*

Risk Rating

   *Significant risk, discuss with doctor immediately

EARLY SIGNS OF UROGENITAL DYSFUNCTION
Urinary Signs

Check each factor that describes you.

_____ You leak urine when coughing, laughing, sneezing, or lifting.*

_____ You have strong urges to urinate, with leaking of urine before getting to the bathroom.*

_____ You urinate frequently during the day.*

_____ You urinate frequently at night.*

_____ You leak urine during sex.*

_____ You wear pads to protect your clothing from urine leakage.*

_____ You feel pain on urination.*

_____ You are unable to empty your bladder completely.*

Risk Rating

   *Significant risk, discuss with doctor immediately

EARLY SIGNS OF UROGENITAL DYSFUNCTION
Sexual Signs
Check each factor that describes you.

_____ You are generally dissatisfied with your sex life.*

_____ You have noticed a sexual problem.*

_____ Your interest in having sex has decreased.*

_____ You have sex less frequently than you used to.*

_____ You feel less pleasure from sexual experience than you used to.*

_____ Your orgasm is less pleasurable.*

_____ You feel pain during intercourse.*

_____ You are unable to achieve orgasm.*

The best indicator of sexual dysfunction is the occurrence of change from previous sexual functioning.

Risk Rating

*Significant risk, discuss with doctor immediately

Besides hormonal factors, there are many other recognized causes of diminished sexual functioning in menopausal women. A few of the most common reasons for midlife women to experience loss of libido are:

- Aging: if a woman has had a low sex drive prior to menopause, it will diminish more during and after menopause
- Medications: many drugs prescribed for psychiatric and general medical illness significantly interfere with sexual functioning.
- Life stressors: being overwhelmed by a mass of personal and professional responsibilities causes stress, anxiety, and depression, all of which diminish the ability to find pleasure in much of anything.

- Substance abuse: taking many drugs for a variety of symptoms, increasing dosages of prescribed medications without medical supervision, ingesting multiple over-the-counter medications simultaneously, and drinking alcohol are all on the rise in women. Interestingly, alcohol consumption increases a woman's risk for promiscuity (and sexually transmitted diseases), but decreases the experience of pleasure during sexual activity.

Most women realize that the experience of pleasure in sexual activities is mostly due to feelings of emotional well-being and pleasure with our partners and less due to the physical pleasure of the act itself. One woman described her orgasms to me as "90 percent my mood and 10 percent my body's response."

How do you feel? Is the overall quality of your life affecting your sexual functioning?

Chapter 16

Osteopenia and Osteoporosis

Osteopenia is low bone mass and osteoporosis is severely reduced bone mass with deterioration of the skeleton and significantly increased risk of fractures.

For women, bone loss begins in our thirties and continues throughout the rest of our lives. By age fifty, half of all women have low bone mass (osteopenia). Even though osteoporosis rates will vary with age, nearly half of all Caucasian women over age fifty will suffer a fracture due to osteoporosis over the course of their lifetime; we don't yet know the prevalence of osteoporotic fractures in non-Caucasian women. Twenty-five million Americans are affected with osteoporosis and 80 percent of them are women. Fractures are often the first sign that the disease has progressed; these fractures cause little pain, so the disease progresses quietly. The fractures that result from this disease are a major cause of disability in women older than fifty. Our most rapid bone loss occurs within the first two to three years before menopause and three to four years after menopause, representing a 5 to 10 percent loss of our bone mass.

During menopause, the greatest bone loss occurs in the spine, hips, and ribs (our weight-bearing bones). Calcium loss in these bones ultimately leads to fractures and pain. The incidence of falls and hip fractures in older women has been steadily increasing every year for the past twenty years, in part due to accelerated bone loss in sedentary older females.

Preventing bone loss involves more than just taking calcium supplements. It involves:

- exercising at least three hours weekly (which can actually increase bone mass);
- eliminating soda from your diet (the phosphates in sodas leach calcium out of the bones);
- adding vitamin and mineral supplements daily (because dietary calcium needs magnesium and other vitamins to be absorbed); and
- starting to take calcium supplements prior to menopause (the higher your bone density prior to menopause, the lower your risk for osteoporosis). The prevention dosage is 600–1,200 mg of calcium per day.

Even in combination with HRT, calcium supplements only reduce the rate of bone loss (prevent thinning). More specific medical treatments are needed if osteoporosis has already occurred.

Even though osteoporosis is more prevalent in Caucasian and Asian women, African-American women are not immune to it and have a delayed onset due normally to larger bones and a tendency to be overweight rather than underweight.

OSTEOPENIA AND OSTEOPOROSIS RISK ASSESSMENT

Non-Changeable Risk Factors
Check each factor that describes you.

    _____ You are older than fifty.*

    _____ You have a family history of osteoporosis.*

_____ You are thin and have a small frame.*

_____ You had an early menopause (before the age of forty).*

_____ You have had a fracture after age fifty.*

_____ You are already being treated for thyroid disease.*

_____ You have had small bowel surgery with resection.*

_____ You have never been pregnant.*

Risk Rating

*Significant risk, discuss with doctor immediately

OSTEOPENIA AND OSTEOPOROSIS RISK ASSESSMENT

Changeable Risk Factors

Check each factor that describes you.

_____ You are an African-American woman who is sixty or older, obese, and you have a poor diet.*

_____ Your diet is low in calcium.*

_____ You are taking medications such as steroids, anticonvulsants, or tranquilizers.*

_____ You are physically inactive.*

_____ You have anorexia or bulimia.

_____ You weigh less now than you did at age twenty-five.

_____ You have more than three caffeinated drinks a day.

_____ You smoke.

_____ You have more than two alcoholic beverages a day.

Risk Rating

Less than three checks: Insignificant risk, no action needed at this time

Three or more checks: Low to moderate risk, discuss with doctor at next exam

*Significant risk, discuss with doctor immediately

EARLY SIGNS OF OSTEOPOROSIS

Check each factor that describes you.

_____ You have lost more than 1.5 inches of height during the postmenopause years.*

_____ You have had a fracture of your wrist, spine, or hip after age fifty.*

_____ Your upper back is curved forward.*

_____ You have chronic pain in the middle of the back (between vertebrae T12 and L1).*

_____ You have osteopenia verified by an ultrasound bone density screening test.*

Risk Rating

*Significant risk, discuss with doctor immediately

Because this disease is painless, fractures discovered on X-ray are often the first indicators of the presence of this disease.

Chapter 17

Thyroid Disease

The thyroid gland is important because it controls and regulates all the chemical and physical changes in our bodies. The thyroid gland needs estrogen to function, and abnormal functioning occurs with estrogen deficiency; it is commonly misdiagnosed as other medical problems. Thyroid disorders are seen predominantly in women, affecting 10 percent of all women over the age of fifty. Currently, twenty million women are being treated for thyroid problems and an estimated two million more are undiagnosed. Thyroid disease is known as "the great imitator." The symptoms are very similar to perimenopause symptoms, and the symptoms usually develop early in life. They are often overlooked during the change of life and can go untreated for many years. Thyroid disease can imitate many illnesses, such as major depression, heart disease, arthritis, and even cancer.

There are many common symptoms suffered by women who are perimenopausal or depressed or have low-functioning thyroid glands (and, occasionally, I've met women with all three disorders occurring simultaneously). Some of these overlapping symptoms are irregular periods, moodiness and irritability, trouble sleeping, fatigue, decreased concentration, short-term memory loss, lack of sexual desire, and weight gain.

There are several thyroid disorders: hyperthyroidism involves an overactive gland and affects 2 percent of all women with thyroid dysfunction; hypothyroidism involves an underactive gland and affects the majority of women with this disorder; and, lastly, thyroid cancer, which is very rare but affects fourteen thousand women yearly.

Current Concepts

Hypothyroidism is the condition resulting from an underactive thyroid.

Thyroid disease is commonly overlooked in perimenopausal women experiencing symptoms of moodiness, sleep disturbance, excessive sweating, and change in the menstrual cycle. This is because so many of the symptoms of perimenopause and thyroid dysfunction overlap with each other (as well as with the symptoms of depression). Sometimes the blood tests for thyroid functioning are borderline normal in women experiencing what are symptoms of thyroid dysfunction. Hence, in practice, if a woman is not responding well to medications for her mood disorder (depression), I will recommend a trial of low-dose thyroid medication to try to determine if the thyroid is the underlying problem.

The thyroid gland needs estrogen to function properly and, during the change of life, borderline thyroid functioning can develop into full-blown thyroid disease. Routine thyroid testing of women being treated for persistent perimenopausal symptoms or depression (and perhaps a trial of low-dose thyroid medication) would help pinpoint the problem.

THYROID DISEASE RISK ASSESSMENT

Non-Changeable Risk Factors

Check each factor that describes you.

_____ You are over fifty years of age.*

_____ You have Type I diabetes (juvenile).*

_____ You have immune system abnormalities (for example, rheumatoid arthritis, lupus, chronic fatigue syndrome, fibromyalgia, or endometriosis).*

_____ You have a family history of thyroid disease.*

_____ You have vitiligo (loss of skin pigmentation).

_____ You have pernicious anemia.

_____ You have prematurely graying hair.

_____ You have been exposed to head and neck irradiation.

Risk Rating

Less than three checks: Insignificant risk, no action needed at this time

Three or more checks: Low to moderate risk, discuss with doctor at next exam

*Significant risk, discuss with doctor immediately

THYROID DISEASE RISK ASSESSMENT

Changeable Risk Factors

Check each factor that describes you.

_____ You are pregnant and have immune system abnormalities.*

_____ Your blood chemistry testing shows an iodine deficiency.*

_____ Your diet is poor in foods rich with vitamins A, C, or E (see part V).*

_____ You take thyroid medication to lose weight (not for thyroid disease).*

_____ You frequently suffer from viral infections.

_____ You are being treated with lithium.

_____ You smoke.

Risk Rating

Less than three checks: Insignificant risk, no action needed at
this time

Three or more checks: Low to moderate risk, discuss with doctor
at next exam

*Significant risk, discuss with doctor immediately

EARLY SIGNS OF THYROID DISEASE

Hyperthyroidism

Check each factor that describes you.

_____ You have unintentionally lost weight recently.*

_____ You are bothered by heart palpitations and periods of racing
heartbeat.*

_____ Your neck has become enlarged.*

_____ You have insomnia.

_____ You get hot flashes.

_____ You have lost your sex drive (this occurs in 50 percent of
affected women).

_____ You suffer from chronic diarrhea.

Risk Rating

Less than three checks: Insignificant risk, no action needed at
this time

Three or more checks: Low to moderate risk, discuss with doctor at next exam

*Significant risk, discuss with doctor immediately

EARLY SIGNS OF THYROID DISEASE

Hypothyroidism

Check each factor that describes you.

_____ You suffer from fatigue and weakness.*

_____ You have menstrual irregularities.*

_____ You are infertile.*

_____ You have lost your sex drive (this occurs in 90 percent of affected women).*

_____ You have elevated cholesterol, as shown by laboratory testing.*

_____ You are gaining weight.

_____ You have thinning hair.

_____ You are irritable.

_____ You have trouble concentrating.

_____ You suffer from constipation.

_____ You suffer from depression.

Risk Rating

Less than four checks: Insignificant risk, no action needed at this time

Four or more checks: Low to moderate risk, discuss with doctor at next exam

*Significant risk, discuss with doctor immediately

Chapter 18

Diabetes

There are two types of diabetes. Type I is a genetic disorder that appears in childhood and is known as juvenile diabetes. Type II is a metabolic disorder of adulthood resulting from the body's inability to properly use its insulin; 95 percent of all diabetics are Type II.

The increasing numbers of new diabetics is becoming an epidemic: more than half of all adult women are overweight; eight million women have diabetes already; and nine out of ten of these women could have prevented the disease with weight loss and lifestyle changes. Unfortunately, most women with this disease don't know they have it because there are no early warning signs, only signs of established disease. Steady, chronic weight gain is a precursor but not an early warning sign.

Diabetes is a serious problem. The medical community now considers it a symptom of cardiovascular disease, which means that *heart disease, heart attack, and stroke are inevitable consequences of diabetes if it is not controlled.* Kidney disease, blindness, and amputation are also disabling consequences of diabetes.

Current Concepts

Insulin resistance syndrome (IRS) is a disease process with abnormal fasting blood glucose test results in middle-aged women. Women of color have a high risk for developing this disease throughout adulthood. It can progress silently into Type II diabetes in the perimenopause years. All overweight women at the onset of perimenopause should be tested for prediabetes status, but you don't have to be overweight to have elevated blood sugar levels. Type II diabetes can lead to heart attack, stroke, and kidney disease. Therefore, it's important to know your risk factors. These are (by physical examination and laboratory tests):

- BMI over 25
- Blood pressure over 130/85
- Fasting glucose over 110 mg/dl
- HDL cholesterol less than 50 mg/dl
- Triglycerides over 150 mg/dl

The American Diabetes Association has published the following warning signs of diabetes:

- Frequent urination
- Excessive thirst
- Weight loss
- Fatigue
- Blurred vision
- Leg pains
- Chronic yeast infections

Visit the website of the American Diabetes Association for more information: www.diabetes.org.

TYPE II DIABETES RISK ASSESSMENT

Non-Changeable Risk Factors

Check each factor that describes you.

_____ You are over forty-five years old.*

_____ You have a family history of diabetes.*

_____ You have polycystic ovarian syndrome.*

_____ You have suffered from gestational diabetes.

_____ One or more of your babies weighed more than nine pounds at birth.

Risk Rating

No checks: Insignificant risk, no action needed at this time

One or more checks: Low to moderate risk, discuss with doctor
at next exam

*Significant risk, discuss with doctor immediately

TYPE II DIABETES RISK ASSESSMENT

Changeable Risk Factors

Check each factor that describes you.

_____ You have impaired glucose tolerance, as shown by laboratory testing.*

_____ You have elevated blood sugar, as shown by screening or laboratory testing.*

_____ You are overweight.*

_____ You are physically inactive.*

_____ You have elevated cholesterol and triglycerides, as shown by laboratory testing.*

_____ You have hypertension, as shown by two or more elevated blood pressure readings.*

_____ You have a poor diet, high in starches and sugars.*
_____ You smoke.

Risk Rating

No checks: Insignificant risk, no action needed at this time

One check: Low to moderate risk, discuss with doctor at next exam

*Significant risk, discuss with doctor immediately

SIGNS OF ESTABLISHED TYPE II DIABETES

Check each factor that describes you.

_____ You have frequent urination.*

_____ You have excessive thirst.*

_____ You have had recent unintentional weight loss and muscle wasting.*

_____ You have blurred vision.

_____ You suffer from fatigue.

_____ You have leg pain and itching.

_____ You have numbness and tingling in your hands and feet.

_____ You have slow healing of cuts and bruises.

_____ You have chronic vaginal yeast infections.

Risk Rating

Less than three checks: Insignificant risk, no action needed at this time

Three or more checks: Low to moderate risk, discuss with doctor at next exam

*Significant risk, discuss with doctor immediately

Chapter 19

Osteoarthritis

Osteoarthritis is a degenerative disease of joint cartilage with breakdown of the cartilage causing pain, limited movement, and bone spurs. Twenty-one million Americans have it, which includes 25 percent of all perimenopausal and postmenopausal women. By the age of sixty-five, two-thirds of women will have X-ray evidence of it whether or not we have symptoms. Therefore, this is a chronic disease of aging. For many of us, it is a source of daily chronic pain. The joints most affected are hands, knees, feet, hips, and spine. Joint pain increases with physical activity, thereby causing most of the disability experienced with this disorder. With pain, our risks increase for depression, agitation, decreased physical activity, and poor sleep and diet. Overall, the disabling pain of osteoarthritis often decreases the quality of one's life.

OSTEOARTHRITIS RISK ASSESSMENT

Non-Changeable Risk Factors

Check each factor that describes you.

_____ You are forty years of age or more.*

_____ You have been overweight for ten or more years.*

_____ You have a family history of diabetes.*

_____ You have a family history of osteoarthritis.*

_____ You have had a joint injury to your knee, hip, or spine.*

_____ You have had infections in your joints.

_____ You have congenital hip disease(s).

_____ You have poor circulation in your hands and feet.

Risk Rating

One check: Insignificant risk, no action needed at this time

Two or more checks: Low to moderate risk, discuss with doctor
at next exam

*Significant risk, discuss with doctor immediately

OSTEOARTHRITIS RISK ASSESSMENT

Changeable Risk Factors

Check each factor that describes you.

_____ You are physically inactive.

_____ Your diet is poor.

_____ You drink less than eight 8-ounce glasses of water daily.

Risk Rating

One check: Insignificant risk, no action needed at this time

Two or more checks: Low to moderate risk, discuss with doctor
at next exam

*Significant risk, discuss with doctor immediately

EARLY SIGNS OF OSTEOARTHRITIS

Check each factor that describes you.

_____ You have morning pain and stiffness in the affected
joints.*

_____ Your pain worsens with use of your joints.*

_____ You have limited motion in the affected joints.*

_____ You have tenderness and swelling in the affected joints.

_____ You have a grating sensation of bone rubbing on bone.

_____ There is a formation of bony knobs at the affected joints.

Risk Rating

One check: Insignificant risk, no action needed at this time

Two or more checks: Low to moderate risk, discuss with doctor
at next exam

*Significant risk, discuss with doctor immediately

Chapter 20

Cancer

Women in the transitional years are afraid of getting cancer. Luckily, the risks aren't high for cancer during these years.

The most common cancers in women are lung, breast, colon, and uterine. Less common are two other uniquely female cancers, cervical and ovarian. Cervical cancer is common but rarely causes death. Ovarian cancer is one of the rarest forms of all cancers, but it almost always causes death. Cancers of the breast, uterus, cervix, and ovaries (the female genital organs) strike fear in the hearts of women because these organs, especially the breast, are a feature of femininity and part of our sexual identity.

The most important issues about cancer are:

- Cancer is not a high-risk disease in perimenopause, but it can't be ignored as a possibility.
- Many of the risk factors for cancer can be altered, but it is best to start changing in your younger years while there is still plenty of time.
- Many cancers have screening techniques for early detection.
- Certain body signs and symptoms can tip you off to a potential problem, and knowing these can save your life.

These six cancers are the ones of greatest concern for women. Following is a brief review of them, their detection methods, and their current treatments.

Lung cancer is the number one cause of cancer death in women. More women die of it than all the other cancers combined. There are no early signs; a means of early detection is being researched currently. There is no effective treatment for this disease and it almost always results in death. The Surgeon General has determined that smoking can be hazardous to your health. Need I say more?

Breast cancer is the second most common cancer in women. Your odds of developing it have been reported as one in eight. This is an average figure, and is true if you are older than eighty-five and have a life expectancy of ninety. See the chart following this discussion. Generally, the odds of developing breast cancer increase as you age. There is a genetic form that comprises 10 percent of all breast cancer. This can be detected by the presence of two cancer genes (BRCA1 and BRCA2) and suspected if your mother or sister has had breast cancer. However, 90 percent of all breast cancer is not genetic and is due to other risk factors. Early detection is the major key to surviving breast cancer, and the breast lumps you find on self-examination can be an early symptom. Breast cancer screening is done by mammography, ultrasound, and magnetic resonance imaging (MRI). You should start having mammograms yearly at age forty. There are many treatments for breast cancer. One is Tamoxifen, a weak estrogen, which is used as a follow-up treatment in women after they have undergone surgery and/or chemotherapy. Tamoxifen is preventive and it lowers the risk of your cancer reappearing.

Colon cancer is the third most common cancer killer of women. While the overall risk of developing this disease is not high, it occurs most commonly in the postmenopausal years. It sometimes develops in thirty- to forty-year-old women with a family history of it. Early detection is made by colonoscopy, which you should have done at age fifty and repeated every five years thereafter. Prevention is accomplished by dietary changes, exercise, and a daily dose of one aspirin.

Colon cancer is more common in women than in men and peaks in incidence between the ages of sixty and seventy-five years. The death rate from this cancer has fallen in the last twenty years because of better and earlier detection, but it remains the third leading cause of cancer deaths in women.

Uterine cancer is the fourth most common cancer in women. It is primarily a disease of postmenopausal women. Detection is by ultrasound and tissue sampling of the uterine lining. Any abnormal uterine bleeding is a trigger for screening for uterine cancer, particularly in the postmenopausal woman. If present, it is always treated with surgery.

Cervical cancer is a young woman's disease and in most cases occurs prior to menopause. The best early detection method is the PAP smear; you should start having one every year at age eighteen. Treatment is cauterization or surgical removal of the cancerous lesion.

Ovarian cancer is the least common of all cancers (only fifteen women out of one hundred thousand will develop it). And it's also the most deadly, with no early warning signs and no early means of detection. It occurs predominantly in women in their sixties and our risks for getting it decrease with advancing age.

Medical research considers both non-modifiable and modifiable risk factors equally important in cancer risk and prevention. If you have *any* risk factors for a cancer type, you are at risk for that cancer as you age. Therefore, all risk factors in the risk assessments that follow are starred because both individually and as a group they are significant. Only if you have *no* risk factors is your disease risk insignificant.

ODDS OF DEVELOPING BREAST CANCER BY AGE

By age 25	1 in 19,608
By age 30	1 in 2,525
By age 35	1 in 622
By age 40	1 in 217
By age 45	1 in 93
By age 50	1 in 50
By age 55	1 in 33
By age 60	1 in 24
By age 65	1 in 17
By age 70	1 in 14
By age 75	1 in 11
By age 80	1 in 10
By age 85	1 in 9
Lifetime	1 in 8

LUNG CANCER RISK ASSESSMENT

Check each factor that describes you.

Non-Changeable Risk Factors

_____ You have a chronic lung disease, for example, emphysema, asthma, chronic bronchitis.*

Changeable Risk Factors

_____ You smoke.*

_____ You are regularly exposed to secondhand smoke.*

_____ You have a diet high in fats.*

_____ You are exposed to a lot of pollutants and carcinogens.*

Risk Rating

No checks: Insignificant risk, no action needed at this time

*Significant risk, discuss with doctor immediately

BREAST CANCER RISK ASSESSMENT

Check each factor that describes you.

Non-Changeable Risk Factors

_____ You have a family history of breast cancer.*

_____ You carry the cancer gene, as shown by genetic screening.*

_____ You have had an abnormal breast biopsy.*

_____ You began to menstruate prior to age thirteen.*

_____ You delivered your first live birth after age thirty.*

_____ Your menopause occurred after age fifty-five.*

_____ You have been receiving estrogen replacement therapy for more than ten years.*

Changeable Risk Factors

_____ You smoke.*

_____ You are obese.*

_____ You have more than two alcoholic beverages a day.*

_____ You are physically inactive.*

_____ You have never been pregnant.*

Risk Rating

No checks: Insignificant risk, no action needed at this time

*Significant risk, discuss with doctor immediately

COLON CANCER RISK ASSESSMENT

Check each factor that describes you.

Non-Changeable Risk Factors

_____ You have a family history of colon cancer.*

_____ You have had a colonoscopy that revealed colon polyps.*

Changeable Risk Factors

_____ You have a diet high in animal fat and low in fiber.*

_____ You are physically inactive.*

_____ You are exposed to a lot of environmental pollutants and carcinogens.*

Risk Rating

No checks: Insignificant risk, no action needed at this time

*Significant risk, discuss with doctor immediately

UTERINE CANCER RISK ASSESSMENT

Check each factor that describes you.

Non-Changeable Risk Factors

_____ You have polycystic ovarian syndrome.*

_____ You have a family history of uterine cancer.*

_____ You have diabetes.*

_____ You have hypertension.*

Changeable Risk Factors

_____ You are receiving estrogen replacement therapy without the addition of progesterone.*

_____ You are obese.*

_____ You smoke.*

Risk Rating

No checks: Insignificant risk, no action needed at this time

*Significant risk, discuss with doctor immediately

CERVICAL CANCER RISK ASSESSMENT

Check each factor that describes you.

Non-Changeable Risk Factors

_____ You are not yet forty years old.*

_____ You have had several abnormal PAP smears.*

_____ You have a family history of cervical cancer.*

Changeable Risk Factors

_____ A sexually transmitted disease, for example, HIV or human papillomavirus, is present in your body.*

_____ You have many sexual partners.*

_____ You engage in unprotected sex.*

Risk Rating

No checks: Insignificant risk, no action needed at this time

*Significant risk, discuss with doctor immediately

OVARIAN CANCER RISK ASSESSMENT

Check each factor that describes you.

Non-Changeable Risk Factors

_____ You have a family history of ovarian cancer.*

_____ You carry the cancer gene, as shown by genetic screening.*

Changeable Risk Factors

_____ You have a uterus and are taking estrogen without progesterone.*

Risk Rating

No checks: Insignificant risk, no action needed at this time

*Significant risk, discuss with doctor immediately

EARLY SIGNS OF CANCER

Check each factor that describes you.

_____ You have discovered breast lumps on self-examination (breast cancer).*

_____ You have had positive findings on a mammography (breast cancer).*

_____ You have had changes in your bowel habits (colon cancer and ovarian cancer).*

_____ You have had blood in your stool (colon cancer).*

_____ You have had polyps found on colonoscopy (colon cancer).*

_____ You have had abnormal vaginal bleeding during your post-menopausal years (uterine cancer and ovarian cancer).*

_____ You have had positive findings on a PAP smear (cervical cancer).*

_____ You have had a positive finding for BRCA1 and BRCA2 on genetic testing (breast cancer).*

_____ You have pelvic pain and/or abdominal pain, bloating, or swelling (uterine cancer and ovarian cancer).*

*Significant risk, discuss with doctor immediately

Chapter 21

Alzheimer's Disease

Alzheimer's disease is a form of dementia. Dementia is a degenerative process of the brain causing slow, progressive loss of mental function, specifically: deterioration in thinking, behavior, mood, and physical and social functioning. It is the most common dementia in the elderly. Alzheimer's is three times more prevalent in women than in men. More than 10 percent of sixty-five-year-old women and more than 50 percent of women older than eighty-five have it. Yet this condition is underdiagnosed and undertreated. The multiple factors that cause this condition are largely unknown.

Memory loss and forgetfulness are a normal part of aging. Alzheimer's involves more than memory problems. It involves the presence of mild cognitive impairments (MCIs). Mild cognitive impairment and memory problems can be detected in your early fifties, and 30 percent to 50 percent of all people who have these symptoms at that age will eventually develop Alzheimer's disease.

ALZHEIMER'S DISEASE RISK ASSESSMENT
Non-Changeable Risk Factors
Check each factor that describes you.

_____ You have a family history of Alzheimer's disease.*

_____ You have had a stroke.*

_____ You have been diagnosed with atherosclerosis (you have cholesterol plaque in your arteries).*

_____ You are sixty-five or older.*

_____ You have had a head injury.*

_____ You have hypertension.*

_____ You have diabetes.*

Risk Rating

No checks: Insignificant risk, no action needed at this time

*Significant risk, discuss with doctor immediately

ALZHEIMER'S DISEASE RISK ASSESSMENT

Changeable Risk Factors

Check each factor that describes you.

_____ You have high cholesterol, as shown by laboratory testing.*

_____ You are obese.*

_____ You smoke.*

_____ You suffer from depression.*

_____ You are physically inactive.

_____ You are mentally inactive.

_____ You are socially isolated.

Risk Rating

No checks: Insignificant risk, no action needed at this time

One to three checks: Low to moderate risk, discuss with doctor at next exam

*Significant risk, discuss with doctor immediately

EARLY SIGNS OF ALZHEIMER'S DISEASE

Check each factor that describes you.

_____ You find it hard to cook meals, pay bills, or use the VCR or DVD player.*

_____ You misplace things and find them in unusual places.*

_____ You are unable to balance your checkbook.*

_____ You are more suspicious and anxious than usual.*

_____ You forget what day it is or often get lost.*

_____ You have lost interest in things you used to enjoy.*

_____ You are usually agitated when making choices and decisions.*

_____ You have become more forgetful of appointments, names, and phone numbers.

_____ You lose your train of thought while talking and forget common words.

_____ You lose your concentration while reading.

Risk Rating

No Checks: Insignificant risk, no action needed at this time

One to three checks: Low to moderate risk, discuss with doctor at next exam

*Significant risk, discuss with doctor immediately

Current Concepts

Many perimenopausal women become fearful that they might have dementia when they experience increasing forgetfulness. I know that I pride myself on being a multitasker, and in the mornings while getting ready for work, my forgetfulness was seriously slowing me down and raising my anxiety about my health.

Researchers from Harvard's School of Public Health tell us that forgetting is normal and that there are several types of forgetfulness, all of which occur with aging but none of which are signs of dementia. These are:

- Transient: forgetting unused facts and events over time;
- Absentminded: the misplacing of something or the forgetting to do something as the result of not paying attention and not focusing on the task at hand;
- Blockage: the inability to recall a name or date, usually due to an overload of other kinds of mental activity, such as thinking about several things at the same time;
- Misattribution: the misplacement or growing inaccuracy of facts because memories grow old as we grow old.

I'm still at my forgetful worst in the morning, but now I don't think I'm losing it. I use notes and reminders to trigger my memory and lots of humor to minimize my frustration.

Chapter 22

Stress and Depression

Depression is twice as prevalent in women as in men, and women are most vulnerable to the onset of depression during their childbearing years. There is an increased prevalence of depression during perimenopause (ages thirty-five to fifty-two). Perimenopause is also likely to be a precipitant for the recurrence of other, preexisting psychiatric illnesses, such as anxiety disorders.

Since depression and anxiety are the most common of all the psychiatric disorders, they are widely researched. Even so, we still don't know why women are twice as susceptible to these disorders as men. Many risk factors have been identified and studied. Stress stands out as the single most important risk factor for developing these disorders.

How many stress symptoms are you experiencing? Use the Stress Symptom Inventory that follows. Pay particular attention to the mental and emotional symptoms because these are the precursors to depression and anxiety disorders. Stress symptoms are intense but brief; they are the reactions to the things we can't control in our lives. However, if the stressors become persistent and chronic, so do the symptoms, and mental illness can develop.

In this chapter, we will handle your risk assessment a little bit differently. First, identify your stress triggers by assessing your current level of satisfaction. Use the form following the Stress Symptom Inventory and score yourself. Then, on the next form, list your current specific stressors and rate each as either positive, negative, or a combination of the two. If you score at medium to low level of satisfaction, you are at risk for developing depression symptoms or, at the very least, your life is unhappy.

I specialize in depression in my psychiatric practice. I've never met a depressed woman who wasn't experiencing life stressors. When I ask my patients what they think caused their psychiatric symptoms, they cite a variety of stressors in their lives as contributing factors. These stress assessments are available on the Internet—I didn't invent them. I've reproduced them for this book to place them in context as precursors of those psychiatric illnesses that are so common in women.

How can you tell the difference between being depressed and just being sad? A list of some distinguishing features follows the list of current specific stressors. Do you have any of these? Are you sad or depressed?

Finally, there are lists of signs and symptoms of the psychiatric syndromes of anxiety and depression. Are you symptomatic?

Stress Symptom Inventory

Think of several times when you have experienced excessive stress and check any of the symptoms you experienced during those times of high stress.

PHYSICAL SYMPTOMS

__Appetite change

__Increase of accidents

__Rash

__Colds/flu

__Increased alcohol, drug, or tobacco use

__Restlessness

__Digestive upsets

__Teeth grinding

__Fatigue

__Insomnia

__Tension

__Finger-drumming, foot-tapping, etc.

__Irregular breathing, hyperventilation

__Weight change

__Pounding heart

__Frequent sighing

__Muscle aches

__Yawning

__Headaches

__Others:_____

_____

MENTAL SYMPTOMS

__Boredom

__Lethargy

__"Weird" or morbid thoughts

__Confusion

__Low productivity

__Difficulty in thinking clearly

__Negative attitude

__Whirling mind

__Poor memory

__Dull senses

__Reduced ability to concentrate

__Forgetfulness

__Others:_____

_____

EMOTIONAL SYMPTOMS

__Anxiety

__Increased use of profanity, put-downs, or sarcasm

__Pessimism

__Bad dreams or nightmares

__Mood swings

__Increased emotionalism

__Nervous laugh

__Crying spells

__Irritability

__Short temper

__Depression

__Little joy

__The "blues"

__Discouragement

__Others:

_____

SPIRITUAL SYMPTOMS

__Apathy

__Loss of faith

__Lowered sex drive

__Cynicism

__Loss of meaning

__Nagging

__Doubt

__Martyrdom

__Resentment

__Emptiness

__Need to "prove" self

__Inability to forgive

__"No one cares" attitude

__Loss of direction

__Others:_____

_____

RELATIONAL SYMPTOMS

__Avoidance of people

__Increased arguing/ disagreements

__Blaming

__Intolerance

__Distrust

__Lack of intimacy

__Fewer contacts with friends

__Lashing out

__Less loving and trusting

ASSESSING YOUR CURRENT LEVEL OF STRESS

Rate your current level of satisfaction

4=Definitely True   3=Somewhat True   2=Neutral or Unsure

1=Mostly Untrue   0=Definitely Untrue

Work/Career

_____ The work I do is challenging.

_____ I have adequate responsibility.

_____ The work I do suits my ability and skills.

_____ The people I work with are supportive.

_____ I have reasonable authority to make decisions.

Money

_____ My job/career meets my financial needs.

_____ My lifestyle is comfortable.

_____ I am able to save a reasonable amount of money.

_____ My spouse/partner is comfortable with our income level.

_____ I am preparing adequately for retirement.

_____ I am comfortable with my/our current level of spending.

Personal

_____ There is someone in my life in whom I can confide almost anything.

_____ I enjoy my social life.

_____ I have friends outside my immediate family with whom I occasionally socialize.

_____ My friends and I sometimes share our problems with one another.

_____ I have a relationship of mutual respect with my friends.

_____ I feel comfortable with members of the opposite sex as friends.

_____ I enjoy sex with my partner.

_____ I am satisfied with my marital status (single, married, living with someone).

_____ My partner frequently lets me know s/he cares.

_____ I feel safe disagreeing with my partner.

_____ My partner and I are able to talk through our differences and resolve most of them.

_____ My partner and I share interests and have fun together.

_____ I feel comfortable with my body (size, shape, color).

Home

_____ I enjoy spending a quiet evening at home.

_____ My home is a place where I can relax and be myself.

_____ I have a hobby I enjoy.

_____ My home is a place of serenity and beauty; it nurtures me.

_____ I take pride in my home.

Levity and Quality of Life

_____ I laugh frequently.

_____ I attend movies, plays, or comedy clubs fairly often.

_____ I can and do laugh at myself.

_____ My sense of humor helps me get through difficult times.

_____ I believe I am making a valuable contribution to the world in some way.

_____ I feel needed and appreciated by those who matter to me.

_____ I have a plan for my life and I am following it.

_____ I am usually able to focus on the positives in life, rather than the negatives.

_____ I've lived my life so that if I died tomorrow, I'd feel fulfilled.

Now add all the points together.

Scale:

124+   *High level of satisfaction.*

78–123 *Medium level of satisfaction.*

0–77   *Lower level of satisfaction.* This may be a good time to take a look at ways of raising your level of happiness and harmony.

WHERE DOES OUR STRESS COME FROM?

My Current Specific Stressors

Personal	Environmental	Job/Career
_____	_____	_____
_____	_____	_____
_____	_____	_____
_____	_____	_____
_____	_____	_____
_____	_____	_____
_____	_____	_____
_____	_____	_____
_____	_____	_____

Although we can cite many different sources of stress, we would probably choose to totally eliminate only a small number of them. Some of our stressors are positive. Did you list your positive ones, too? In addition to those we acknowledge as completely positive, others have positive aspects to them. How many of your stressors are combinations (sometimes positive, sometimes negative)? Take a moment to go back and put a (+) next to those that are completely positive and a (-) next to the negative ones. Put both signs next to the combination ones. Many people find that the majority of items on their list are combination stressors.

DIFFERENCES BETWEEN DEPRESSION AND NORMAL SADNESS

Features	Normal Sadness	Depression
____ Recent difficult or tragic life event	Common	Unusual
____ Family history of depression	Absent	Present
____ Mood variation	Depression worse late in the day	Depression worse in the morning
____ Sleep disturbances	Difficulty in falling asleep but remains asleep	Middle of the night or early morning insomnia
____ Appetite	May be increased or decreased; mild or no rapid weight loss	Little interest in food; weight loss
____ Physical ailments	Fewer and less severe	Many and more severe
____ Physical and mental activity	Mild slowing or, more rarely, agitation	Moderate to severe slowing
____ Attitude	Self-pity, pessimism, but no loss of self-esteem	Self-blame, remorse, guilt, complete loss of self-esteem
____ Interest	Mild to moderate loss, but usually able to work	Pervasive loss of interest or pleasure in everything

Source: Reprinted from *Health and Nutrition Newsletter,* (Columbia University School of Public Health) vol. 2, no. 10.

SIGNS OF ANXIETY

Check each factor that describes you.

_____ You are often nervous.*

_____ You have difficulty concentrating.*

_____ You are often afraid.*

_____ You are restless.

_____ You don't sleep well.

_____ You have lost your energy.

_____ You shake, tremble, or wring your hands.

_____ Your heart races or your breathing is fast.

_____ You have chest pains.

_____ You have stomach aches or diarrhea.

_____ Your muscles are tense or painful.

_____ You constantly worry.

Risk Rating

Less than four checks: Insignificant risk, no action needed at this time

Four or more checks: Low to moderate risk, discuss with doctor at next exam

*Significant risk, discuss with doctor immediately

SIGNS OF DEPRESSION

Check each factor that describes you.

_____ You have insomnia or excessive sleeplessness.*

_____ You no longer enjoy activities that once brought you pleasure.*

_____ You have a sense of helplessness and gloom.*

_____ You have recurrent thoughts of suicide and death.*

_____ You have lost your appetite and some weight.

_____ Your energy level is low.

_____ You have lost some of your self-esteem.

_____ Your productivity has fallen.

_____ Your attention span has decreased or you are more frequently confused.

_____ You have withdrawn from social interaction.

_____ You are frequently irritable or angry.

_____ You constantly reproach yourself or feel an inappropriate amount of guilt.

Risk Rating

Less than four checks: Insignificant risk, no action needed at this time

Four or more checks: Low to moderate risk, discuss with doctor at next exam

*Significant risk, discuss with doctor immediately

Now that you have completed part III, go to part III of the MAP and complete it, reflecting your work here.

Part IV

To Be or Not To Be on HRT

Chapter 23

First Thoughts

Hormone replacement therapy isn't a new idea. Researchers have been developing products for the past forty years. In the 1950s and 1960s, estrogen-based drugs were prescribed to prevent miscarriages. In the 1970s and 1980s, oral contraceptives were developed. In the 1990s, safer, more effective, lower-dose birth control pills were developed.

What are the so-called "natural" products we hear about? "Natural" means to exist in nature and "synthetic" means put together or custom-designed. There are no human-derived products. Some, like Premarin, are made from the urine of pregnant horses. Others, like estradiol, are made from soy and Mexican yam. All these products started from the same animal or plant materials and were custom-designed in the laboratory.

Hormone replacement therapy (HRT) and estrogen replacement therapy (ERT) have traditionally been prescribed to provide symptom relief during perimenopause, menopause, and surgically induced menopause; to treat physical changes due to permanently low estrogen levels; and to protect against diseases common to women in the postmenopause years. Relief? Treatment? Protection? Sounds good. You may have noticed, however, that not every woman over forty-five is on HRT. That's because all women are not the same and each woman must be evaluated individually. Some of the issues to consider are the kind of symptoms or changes you present, your future disease risk, the form of treatment you prefer, the likely efficacy of HRT for you, as well as your own history and health status.

So, how do you know if it's right for you? Start figuring it out by answering the following questions. We will look at the implications of your answers in the context of your issues, and I want you to raise them with your doctor when you discuss HRT.

CIRCLE YES OR NO
Have you had a total or partial hysterectomy?   Y   N
Have you had chemotherapy or irradiation therapy?   Y   N

Do you have any of these symptoms?
Irregular periods or cessation of periods   (Y)   N
Hot flashes and/or night sweats   (Y)   N
Insomnia   *Sometimes* Y   N
Heart palpitations   Y   N
Irritability   (Y)   N
Decreased sexual libido   Y   N
Depression   (Y)   N
Memory loss   (Y)   N

These are common symptoms that midlife women seek treatment for, and all of these can continue into the postmenopause years. In fact, one in five of us continue to have symptoms after menopause. The FDA has approved the use of HRT to treat menopausal symptoms.

CIRCLE YES OR NO

Are your symptoms worsening?	Ⓨ	N
Have your symptoms persisted after menopause?	Y	N
Did you get your symptoms suddenly after gynecological surgery?	Y	N
Are your symptoms interfering with the quality of your life?	Ⓨ	N
If so, jot down how:_____		

Are you experiencing any of these physical changes?

Vaginal dryness	Ⓨ	N
Pain or bleeding during intercourse	Y	N
Urine leakage (when sneezing, coughing, bending, or lifting)	Y	N
Recurring urinary tract infections	Y	N
Wrinkling skin	Ⓨ	N
Weight gain (with fat accumulation at your waist, hips, and thighs)	Ⓨ	N
Impaired vision (night blindness, increasing farsightedness)	Ⓨ	N
Are these changes worsening?	Ⓨ	N
Are any of these changes interfering with the quality of your life?	Ⓨ	N
If so, jot down how:_____		

Are you at risk for any of these diseases in your later years (refer to part III)?

Osteoporosis (the FDA has approved the use of HRT for the prevention of osteoporosis)	Y	N

Cardiovascular disease	Y	N
Alzheimer's disease	Y	N
Colon cancer	Y	N
Uterine cancer	Y	N
Breast cancer	Y	N

Is prescription medication the way you prefer to cope with physical and/or emotional problems? Women are strongly divided in their preference for treatment. Some prefer prescription medications and management of their symptoms by their doctor. Others prefer nonprescription alternatives. However, all women are concerned about the health implications of long-term use of any product for symptom relief.

Chapter 24

Is it Safe for Me?

HRT can have long-term health risks. If you are going to take HRT, you need to embrace a healthy lifestyle. There are reasons why you shouldn't take it.

Before taking HRT, you should find out the following:

Your blood pressure _____

Your resting pulse rate _____

Your height _____

Your weight _____

Your current body mass index (BMI) _____

Your blood glucose level _____

Your blood cholesterol levels _____

Total cholesterol _____

HDL _____

LDL _____

Triglycerides _____

The results of your PAP smear Normal/Abnormal

The results of your mammogram Normal/Abnormal

Your estrogen level Normal/Low

The result of your bone density screening _____

Your doctor will prescribe the appropriate screenings/tests if you ask. Ask!

Do you know how to do a breast self-examination? Learn. I'll tell you why in the next chapter. You will examine yourself using your sense of touch, familiarizing yourself with your body, and looking for changes.

Are you willing to make some lifestyle changes? I'm referring to stopping smoking, taking vitamins, beginning to exercise, and developing a healthy diet. We'll look at why in part V.

Now we come to what doctors call, "contraindications," or reasons to be cautious in prescribing HRT, or not to prescribe it at all.

HRT should be taken with caution, and by non-oral routes (by injection, by skin patch, etc.), if you have any of the following:
- Elevated blood cholesterol and/or triglycerides
- Endometriosis
- Uterine fibroids
- Gallbladder disease
- Seizures
- Migraine headaches

HRT is not safe to take if you have any of these problems:
- Breast cancer, past or present
- Endometrial cancer in the past five years
- Unexplained vaginal bleeding
- Liver disease
- A history of blood clots
- A blood coagulation disorder, such as sickle-cell trait

Chapter 25

Recent Research Findings and Controversies

The Women's Health Initiative (WHI) is a study of 16,600 healthy women in postmenopause. They have participated in the study for up to five years. The women were divided into two groups: one received HRT and the other received a placebo. The Heart and Estrogen/Progestin Replacement Study (HERS) is a study of twenty-seven hundred postmenopausal women, all of whom had or have Coronary Heart Disease. These women have participated in this study for up to six years. They were also divided into HRT and placebo groups.

Most women who use HRT start at perimenopause or early menopause. In these studies, however, the average age was sixty-five, so the women had been in postmenopause for at least ten years. Menopause/postmenopause can be divided into three stages: early (the first one to three years), intermediate (the next five to ten years), and late (beyond ten years). Each stage is characterized by its physical symptoms and physical changes. Below is an indication of the usefulness of HRT during each stage.

EARLY STAGE

✓Vasomotor symptoms	Hot flashes	
	Night sweats	
	Sleep deprivation	
	Heart palpitations	
✓Mood disorders	Irritability	
	Depressed mood	
Urogenital symptoms	Urinary incontinence	
✓Memory	Short-term memory loss	

USEFULNESS OF HRT

HRT can eliminate or significantly reduce all symptoms except urinary incontinence, which it can worsen; it can also cause resumption of vaginal bleeding

The physical symptoms of early menopause/postmenopause are usually temporary.

INTERMEDIATE STAGE | USEFULNESS OF HRT

Urogenital changes	Uterine fibroids	Can increase their growth
	Urinary tract infections	
Sexual dysfunction	Vaginal dryness	HRT reverses the atrophy that underlies these four changes, reducing their severity
	Vaginal infections	
	Pain/bleeding on intercourse	
✓Skin atrophy	Thinning/drying skin	HRT can reduce and delay these skin and hair changes
	Wrinkles	
	Hair loss	
✓Metabolic changes	Weight gain	Oral HRT can cause gains
	High cholesterol	Can cause increase in LDLs
	Gallstones	Can increase incidence
	Osteopenia	Can reduce bone thinning
	Liver disease	Can elevate liver enzymes
	Blood clotting	Can increase risk of clotting in those with a history
Teeth	Tooth Loss	HRT can eliminate these changes
	Gum disease	

The intermediate stage can include any or all of the early stage physical symptoms as well as those included above.

The **LATE STAGE** is characterized by the development of disease.

USEFULNESS OF HRT

Bone

Osteoporosis	Fractures of the hip and spine	HRT reduces bone thinning and the risk of fractures
	Loss of height	

Heart

Cardiovascular disease	Hypertension	HRT in the first year of use can increase risk in women who have established disease of the arteries
	Athersclerosis	
	Adult-onset diabetes	

Colon

Gastrointestinal disease	Colon polyps	Not studied
	Colon cancer	HRT can decrease this risk

Breast

	Benign breast tumors	Increase in abnormal mammograms in the first year of use
	Breast cancer	Oral HRT use greater than five years can increase risk

Uterus/Bladder/Ovary

	Urogenital disease	Not studied
	Prolapsed bladder	Estrogen replacement therapy taken alone can cause cancer in women who have a uterus
	Uterine cancer	
	Ovarian cancer	Long-term use increases risk

Brain

	Macular degeneration (retinal disease)	Not studied
	Alzheimer's disease	Does not protect against dementia and may increase risk

Most women who take and continue to take HRT have menopausal symptoms that interfere with their quality of life. These two studies did not evaluate whether or not quality of life was improved by HRT.

If you use HRT, the benefits (symptom relief) must outweigh your risks. You should know all your potential risks, and you should use HRT under strict medical supervision.

Recommendations

- Before starting HRT, every woman should have a disease risk assessment for breast cancer, heart disease, blood coagulation disorders, colorectal cancer, osteoporosis, ovarian cancer, and liver and gallbladder disease.
- Consider taking HRT for less than five years to control hot flashes and vaginal dryness.
- All women with a uterus who take estrogen must also have adequate progesterone prescribed to prevent development of uterine cancer.
- HRT should not be prescribed for the prevention of heart disease.
- HRT should not be prescribed as the first choice for prevention of osteoporosis because of its risks with long-term use, i.e., breast cancer, gallbladder disease, exacerbation of heart disease, but it is a good second choice if other treatment has not worked.
- Be prepared to make some lifestyle changes in order to take HRT as safely as possible.

I am cautious about prescribing any medication for an indefinite period of time. Taking medication alone is not a substitute for adopting good health habits. In practice, I try hard to get my patients to institute lifestyle changes in addition to taking medication.

If you are already using HRT medications or are seriously considering using these prescription products, you must be prepared to stop smoking, limit alcohol consumption to one drink a day, and maintain a normal body weight.

Smoking affects the blood vessels in the heart and lungs and, in combination with HRT, which can raise your cholesterol levels, the risk of heart disease goes up dramatically.

Alcohol consumption decreases the functioning of the immune system, can worsen the symptoms of fibrocystic breast disease, and increase your risk for breast cancer by damaging breast cells. And alcohol triggers hot flashes, the very symptom we're trying to treat with HRT. Alcohol consumption also encourages weight gain and it interferes with the absorption of nutrients from our food.

Are you overweight? If you are, I would advise against taking HRT for the following reasons:

- HRT can increase your risks for heart disease and breast cancer if you are susceptible to these.
- Excess body fat increases your susceptibility to these diseases in the postmenopause years.
- Weight gain often leads to obesity, which is a sign of overeating and malnutrition.

Obese women are at risk for osteoporosis because poor nutrition can lead to accelerated bone thinning and bone loss during perimenopause; HRT by itself will not overcome the deleterious effects of poor nutrition on bone mass.

Even short-term use of HRT is under intense scrutiny. HRT has had FDA approval to treat moderate to severe menopausal symptoms such as hot flashes and night sweats. However, changes in breast tissue and abnormal mammograms show up frequently in the first year of HRT use, and HRT has been shown to stimulate the growth of breast cancer cells during short-term use. Overall, studies with estrogen/progestin combination therapies revealed that participating women had an increased risk of breast cancer, heart attacks, blood clots, and strokes after five years of use as compared to women who did not use HRT. Most of these findings apply to combination drugs—those containing both estrogen and progestin. Studies of drugs with estrogen alone are still going on.

If you have been taking HRT and decide to stop taking it, wean yourself off the medication slowly, giving yourself progressively lower doses over several weeks until you reach the zero point. Some of you will get your symptoms back as you stop your medication—vaginal changes, skin changes, hair thinning, and resumption of hot flashes. And, in some of you, these symptoms won't go away.

Overall, HRT is no longer considered the first choice and best treatment for menopause symptoms and prevention of post-menopause disease. If you are taking HRT and want to consider stopping, the following algorithm (decision tree) may help you clarify the issues and options.

Can you treat these symptoms in other ways? Can you take other preventive measures? Chapter 28 will present alternative treatments, as will part V.

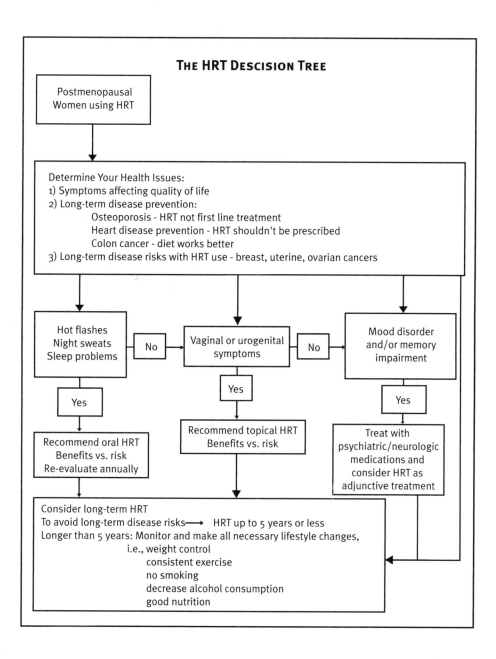

THE HRT DESCISION TREE

Postmenopausal
Women using HRT

Determine Your Health Issues:
1) Symptoms affecting quality of life
2) Long-term disease prevention:
    Osteoporosis - HRT not first line treatment
    Heart disease prevention - HRT shouldn't be prescribed
    Colon cancer - diet works better
3) Long-term disease risks with HRT use - breast, uterine, ovarian cancers

Hot flashes
Night sweats
Sleep problems

No

Vaginal or urogenital
symptoms

No

Mood disorder
and/or memory
impairment

Yes

Yes

Yes

Recommend oral HRT
Benefits vs. risk
Re-evaluate annually

Recommend topical HRT
Benefits vs. risk

Treat with
psychiatric/neurologic
medications and
consider HRT as
adjunctive treatment

Consider long-term HRT
To avoid long-term disease risks⟶ HRT up to 5 years or less
Longer than 5 years: Monitor and make all necessary lifestyle changes,
    i.e., weight control
        consistent exercise
        no smoking
        decrease alcohol consumption
        good nutrition

Chapter 26

What Products Are Out There?

There is a large variety of hormone products currently available.

In addition to increasing your risk for certain diseases such as cancer, these products can cause side effects when taken for either short-term or long-term use. Here's a partial listing of side effects that women most commonly complain about:

- Weight gain, fluid retention, bloating, PMS-like symptoms
- Restarting of the menstrual cycle, breakthrough bleeding, spotting
- Vaginal yeast infections
- Breast enlargement, tenderness, and cystic disease
- Headaches, dizziness, increased migraine attacks
- Fatigue, moodiness, nervousness

This listing is meant to indicate that there are many products available and that you have a range of choices and routes of administration to choose from. If you have a uterus, you must take a progestin with estrogen replacement. For convenience, there are the combination products in oral form. If you've had a hysterectomy, I would recommend you try estrogen replacement in forms other than oral; side effects are more common with oral dosing.

Available Hormone Products*

Alora (estrogen patch)

Amen (progestin/progesterone)

Aygestin (progestin/ progesterone)

Biestrogen (oral estrogen)

Climara (estrogen patch)

CombiPatch (combination estrogen and progesterone)

Crinone (progestin/progesterone)

Cycrin (progestin/progesterone)

Estrace (oral estrogen)

Estrace cream (vaginal estrogen)

Estraderm (estrogen patch)

Estradiol with Progesterone (combination estrogen and progesterone)

Estratab (oral estrogen)

Estratest (testosterone)

Estriol cream (vaginal estrogen)

Estring (vaginal estrogen)

Evista (SERM)

FemHRT (combination estrogen and progesterone)

FemPatch (estrogen patch)

Menest (oral estrogen)

Methyltestosterone (testosterone)

Micronor (progestin/ progesterone)

Natural Micronized Progesterone (progestin/progesterone)

Natural Progesterone Cream (transdermal cream)

Nor-QD (progestin/progesterone)

Ogen (oral estrogen)

Ogen (vaginal estrogen)

Ortho-Est (oral estrogen)

Premarin (oral estrogen)

Premarin (vaginal estrogen)

Premphase (combination estrogen and progesterone)

Prempro (combination estrogen and progesterone)

Pro-Gest body cream (transdermal cream)

Progestasert (vaginal progesterone)

Prometrium (progestin/ progesterone)

Provera (progestin/ progesterone)

Testosterone capsules (testosterone)

Testosterone cream (transdermal cream)

Triestrogen (oral estrogen)

Vivelle (estrogen patch)

*This is a partial listing as of this writing; the pharmaceutical companies continually develop new products and refine methods of delivery.

‎

ORAL ESTROGENS				
Product Name	**Company**	**Doses**	**Est. Cost/Mo.**	**Source**
Premarin (Conjugated estrogens)	Wyeth-Ayerst	0.3 mg, 0.9 mg 0.625 mg, 1.25 mg 2.5 mg/day	$17 - $21	Pregnant mare's urine
Estrace Isomolecular estradiol	Mead-Johnson is a division of Brisol-Myers Squibb	0.5 mg, 2.0 mg, 1.0 mg/day	$13 - $23	Plant-derived
Ortho-Est Isomolecular estrone sulfate (aka estropipate)	Ortho Pharmaceuticals	0.625 mg or 1.25 mg/day	$15 - $19	Plant-derived
Ogen Isomolecular estrone sulfate (aka estropipate)	Pharmacia Upjohn	0.625 mg or 1.25 mg/day	$11 - $14	Plant-derived
Menest (esterified estrogens which are 75-85% isomolecular sodium sulfates—not a human estrogen)	Monarch Pharmaceuticals	0.3 mg, 0.625 mg, 1.25, or 2.5 mg/day	$8 - $22	Plant-derived
Triestrogen Isomolecular estrone, estradiol, estriol	Compounding Pharmacies	1.25 mg 2x day Commonly prescribed for one in A.M. and one in P.M.	$42	Plant-derived
Biestrogen Isomolecular estradiol, estriol	Compounding Pharmacies	1.25 mg 2x day Commonly prescribed for one in A.M. and one in P.M.	$42	Plant-derived

ESTROGEN PATCHES				
Product Name	**Company**	**Doses**	**Est. Cost/Mo.**	**Source**
Estraderm	Ciba-Geigy	.05 or 0.1 mg/day	$24	Plant-derived
Vivelle	Ciba-Geigy	.035, .05, .075, or 0.1 mg/day	$26	Plant-derived
Alora	Proctor & Gamble	.05, .075, or 0.1 mg/day	$25	Plant-derived
Climara	Berlex Laboratories	0.5 or 0.1 mg/day	$25	Plant-derived
FemPatch	Parke-Davis	0.02 mg/day	$29	Plant-derived

PROGESTINS/PROGESTERONE						
Product Name	**Company**	**Doses**	**Est. Cost/Mo**	**Source**	**Equiv. Doses**	**Comments**
Nor-QD (Norethindone)	Syntex	0.35 mg tabs in a 42-day pack	$25/pack	Synthetic	0.70 mg	A progestational birth control pill; continuous treatment causes upset stomach, nausea, and headaches
Micronor (Norethindone)	Ortho Pharmaceuticals	0.35 mg tabs in a 28-day pack	$29/pack	Synthetic	0.70 mg	See above
Aygestin (Norethindone)	Wyeth-Ayerst	0.5 mg	$38	Synthetic	0.625 mg	Potentially up to 10 mg may be used daily for 5-10 days
Provera (medroxy-progesterone acetate abbreviated as MPA)	Pharmacia Upjohn	Continuous: 2.5 mg; Cycled 5.0, or 10.0 mg	$17 - $31	Synthetic	Gold standard for comparison 2.5 mg	Provera is Medroxy-progesterone; effects in some women are dose dependent
Cycrin (MPA)	Wyeth-Ayerst	Continuous: 2.5 mg; Cycled 5.0, or 10.0 mg	$11 - $14		See Provera	See Provera comments
Amen (MPA)	Carnick Laboratories	5.0 or 10.0 mg	$15	Synthetic	See Provera	See Provera comments

HORMONE THERAPY OPTIONS FOR MENOPAUSE						
Product Name	**Company**	**Doses**	**Est. Cost/Mo**	**Source**	**Equiv. Doses**	**Comments**
Natural micronized isomolecular progestrone (NMP) in oil	Compounding Pharmacies	100 mg 2x daily on days 14-28 or 100-300 mg daily for continuous dosing given in divided doses	Varies $35 to $60	Plant-derived	Continuous dose equivalent to approx. 2.5 mg Provera; cycled dose equiv. to appox. 5-10 mg of Provera	PMS Symptoms
Prometnum Isomolecular NMP	Solvay	100 mg daily for continuous dosing given in divided doses	$18 (30 capsules)	Plant-derived	Unknown	Used in Europe and Orient; contraindicated for women with allergy to peanuts
Crinone Isomolecular Progesterone	Wyeth-Ayerst	4% gel delivering 45 mg/applicator 8% gel delivering 90 mg/applicator	at 4% is $30 for the 6 appli-cators used per cycle	Plant-derived	Unknown	Natural progesterone used beginning 15th day of cycle
Progestasert	————	IUD	Annual insertion	Micronyld progest-erone		Slight risk of perforation

COMBINATION ESTROGEN WITH PROGESTIN OR PROGESTERONE

Product Name	Company	Doses	Est. Cost/Mo.	Source
Prempro	Wyeth	Daily doses of Premarin .625 mg MPA 2.5 or 5.0 mg	$22	Pregnant Mare's Urine/ Synthetic
Premphase	Wyeth	Premarin .625 mg for days 1-28 MPA 5.0 mg for days 14-28	$20	Pregnant Mare's Urine/ Synthetic
Estradiol with natural micronized isomolecular progesterone	Compounding Pharmacies	Estradiol 0.5 mg NMP 100 mg 2x daily	$45	Plant-derived
CombiPatch (The only combinaton product with a transderman patch delivery. Other combination products are administered orally.)	Rhone-Poulenc Rorer	Patch contains Estradiol 05 mg and 0.25 mg Norethindrone acetate	$30	Estrogen is plant-derived and isomolecular, projestin is synthetic
FemHRT	Parke-Davis	Estradiol .05 mg Northindrone 1 mg	$35	Estrogen and progestine

VAGINAL ESTROGENS						
Product Name	**Company**	**Doses**	**Est. Cost/Mo**	**Source**	**Equiv. Doses**	**Comments**
Estrace cream Isomolecular estradiol	Mead-Johson (a division of Bristol-Myer)	2 gm every night for 2 weeks then 1 gm 3x week	$36	Plant-derived	0.1 mg estradiol per gram	Lower pH than Premarin
Premarin Conjugated estrogens	Wyeth-Ayerst	0.5 to 2 gm daily for 3 wks w/ 1 wk off	$40	Pregnant mare's urine	0.625 mg per gram	
Esteriol cream Isomolecular estriol	Compounding Pharmacies	0.5 mg vaginally for 21 days then 0.5 mg 2x week	$10	Plant-derived	0.5 per gram	
Ogen Estropipate	Pharmacia Upjohn	2.0 to 4.0 gms daily for 3 weeks with 1 week off	$44	Plant-derived	1.5 mg per gram	
Estring vaginal silicone ring isomolecular estradiol	Pharmacia Upjohn	2 mg delivered over 90 days	$60 for one ring	Plant-derived	Not applicable	Placed in vagina like a diaphragm

TESTOSTERONE				
Product Name	**Company**	**Doses**	**Est. Cost/Mo.**	**Source**
Estratest Esterified estrogens with methyltestosterone Estratest HS	Solvay	1.25 mg estrogen with 2.5 mg testosterone, 0.625 mg estrogen with 1.25 mg testosterone	$30	Plant-derived/synthetic
Testosterone capsules in oil Isomolecular testosterone	Compounding Pharmacy	1.25 mg to 5.0 mg with A.M. dosing	$20	Plant-derived
Methyltestosterone	Compounding Pharmacy	0.125 to 0.8 mg/day	Varies	Synthetic

TRANSDERMAL CREAMS				
Product Name	**Company**	**Doses**	**Est. Cost/Mo.**	**Source**
Estradiol cream Isomolecular estradol	Compounding Pharmacy	0.05 mg/gm to 0.1 mg/gm (1/8 tsp 2x daily)	$10	Plant-derived
Natural progesterone cream Isomolecular progesterone	Compounding Pharmacy	10 to 20 mg of progesterone 2x daily	$30	Plant-derived
*Pro-Gest Body Cream Isomecular progesterone *Included because of widespread nonprescriptive use. Progesterone levels verified by independent laboratory.	Transitions For Health, Inc. Portland, OR 800-888-6814 7A.M.–5P.M. Pacific Time	There are 450 mg of natural progesterone in one ounce of cream— contact company for usage	2.0 oz tube is $31.95 (enough for about 42 1/4 tsp amounts)	Plant-derived
Testosterone cream Isomolecular testosterone	Compounding Pharmacy	0.1 to 0.5 mg/gm	$18	Plant-derived

SELECTIVE ESTROGEN RECEPTOR MODULATOR (SERM)				
Product Name	**Company**	**Doses**	**Est. Cost/Mo.**	**Source**
Evista Raloxifen	Eli Lilly	60 mg daily	$60	Synthetic

©1997 Revised November 1998 by Marla Ahlgrimm, RPh (Women's Health America, Madison, WI); Susan Doughty, CNP (New England Women's Center, Portland, ME); Chris Groth, RPh (St. Luke's Medical Center, Milwaukee, WI); Kayt Klein Havens, MD (U of WI Medical School, Milwaukee, WI), and Ann Kopel, MS (Oregon Menopause Network, Portant, OR); Sarah Ray, PharmD (St. Luke's Medical Center Medical Center). May be reproduced for educational purposes only. First printed as a supplement to *Health Forum Midlife Women*, vol. 3 no. 2 Spring 1997, quarterly newsletter of the Oregon Menopause Network (2607 SE Hawthorne Blvd. Portland, OR 97214 503-232-9446).

The hormone chart has been reproduced by permission from a supplement to *Health Forum for Midlife Women*, vol. 3, no. 2, Spring 1997, quarterly newsletter of the Oregon Menopause Network.

Disclaimer: this chart has been compiled as a public service and in no way represents a recommendation of any product or method of use. The accuracy of the information is not guaranteed. Product prices vary even within the same region of the country. Those who compiled this chart are not responsible for the use of any product listed which should only be used with the advice of a trusted, licensed healthcare provider. It is important to monitor drug levels and therapeutic response since individuals vary. "Isomolecular" notes a hormone with a chemical structure matching humans.

Chapter 27

Your Initial Evaluation and Follow-Up for HRT

The physician guidelines for prescribing HRT are applied inconsistently. I commonly see women who receive a year's prescription for HRT with little scheduled follow-up, if any, during that year. I suppose the assumption is that we'll complain if we see a problem. But women want to use HRT under the safest possible circumstances and feel confident that it's actually meeting their individual needs. I believe a workup and follow-up for prescribing HRT should look like this:

Initial Evaluation
- Screen for disease risks
- Screen for contraindications to use
- Choose reasons for prescribing HRT
- Select a drug
- Emphasize that healthy lifestyle changes must accompany HRT, i.e., weight control, exercise, smoking cessation

Get Baselines
- Body mass index
- Blood pressure
- Blood glucose

- Blood cholesterol
- Routine gynecological examination
- Hormone panel
- Bone mineral density

30-Day Follow-Up
- Assess for changes in body mass index
- Assess for changes in blood pressure
- Assess for changes in blood glucose
- Assess for changes in blood cholesterol after six weeks
- Teach patient how to perform a breast self-examination
- Assess for side effects
- Assess for effectiveness

90-Day Follow-Up
- Assess for changes in body mass index
- Assess for changes in blood pressure
- Assess for changes in blood glucose
- Assess for changes in blood cholesterol
- Ask if patient is performing breast self-examinations
- Ask if patient has modified her diet, begun to exercise, or quit smoking

6-Month Follow-Up
- Repeat 90-Day Follow-Up

1-Year Follow-Up
- Repeat initial workup
- Repeat the initial workup at yearly intervals up to five years, then slowly wean the patient off medication.

ALTERNATIVES FOR SYMPTOM RELIEF, PHYSICAL CHANGES, AND DISEASE PREVENTION			
Herbals and Vitamins	**Symptoms: Hot Flashes**	**Vaginal Dryness**	**Mood Swings/ Insomnia**
Bioflavinoids	✓	✓	
Black Cohosh	✓	✓	✓
Calcium			
Chamomile Tea			✓
Chickweed	✓		
Dandelion	✓		✓
Dong Quai	✓	✓	✓
Elderflower	✓		
Flaxseed		✓	✓
Garden Sage	✓	✓	✓
Ginko Biloba			✓
Ginseng			
Hops	✓		✓
Licorice	✓	✓	✓
Magnesium			
Melatonin			✓
Mexican Wild Yam	✓	✓	✓
Mother Wort	✓	✓	✓
Cat Straw			✓
Phosphorus			
Red Clover	✓		✓
St. John's Wort			✓
Soy	✓	✓	✓
SAMe			✓
Valerian			✓
Ipriflavone			
Vitamin A			
Vitamin B6			✓
Vitamin C			
Vitamin D			
Vitamin E	✓	✓	
Vitamin K			
Zinc			

ALTERNATIVES FOR SYMPTOM RELIEF, PHYSICAL CHANGES, AND DISEASE PREVENTION			
Herbals and Vitamins	**Sexual Dysfunction**	**Prevention**	
		Osteo	**CVD**
Bioflavinoids			
Black Cohosh			
Calcium		✓	✓
Chamomile Tea			
Chickweed			
Dandelion			
Dong Quai			
Elderflower			
Flaxseed			
Garden Sage	✓		
Ginko Biloba			
Ginseng	✓		
Hops			
Licorice			
Magnesium		✓	
Melatonin			
Mexican Wild Yam			
Mother Wort			
Cat Straw			
Phosphorus		✓	
Red Clover			
St. John's Wort			
Soy			
SAMe			✓
Valerian			
Ipriflavone		✓	
Vitamin A		✓	
Vitamin B6		✓	
Vitamin C		✓	
Vitamin D		✓	
Vitamin E			
Vitamin K		✓	
Zinc		✓	

ALTERNATIVES FOR SYMPTOM RELIEF, PHYSICAL CHANGES, AND DISEASE PREVENTION			
Pharmaceuticals	**Symptoms: Hot Flashes**	**Vaginal Dryness**	**Mood Swings**
Antidepressants:	✓		✓
Prozac Dosage: 10-20 mg daily	✓		✓
Paxil CR Dosage: 12.5-25 mg daily	✓		✓
Effevor XR Dosage: 37.5-75 mg daily	✓		✓
Cadiovascular Drugs: Catopress Norvasec	✓ ✓		
Vaginal Lubricants Astroglide, Reptens		✓	
Cholesterol Drugs* (Statin Drugs): Mevacor Zocor Lipotor Lescol Pravochol			
Antihypertension Drugs (Beta Blockers) (Ace Inhibitors) Zasotec			
K-Y Jelly		✓	
Fosomax (Bisphosphonates) (Also Actonel)			
Evista (SERM)			
ASA			
Bellergal	✓		✓
Clonidine	✓		
Lofexidene	✓		
Megace	✓		
Birth Control Pills	✓	✓	✓

ALTERNATIVES FOR SYMPTOM RELIEF, PHYSICAL CHANGES, AND DISEASE PREVENTION			
Pharmaceuticals	**Sexual Dysfunction**	**Prevention**	
		Osteo	**CVD**
Antidepressants: Prozac Dosage: 10-20 mg daily Paxil CR Dosage: 12.5-25 mg daily Effevor XR Dosage: 37.5-75 mg daily			
Cadiovascular Drugs: Catopress Norvasec			
Vaginal Lubricants Astroglide, Reptens	✓		
Cholesterol Drugs* (Statin Drugs): Mevacor Zocor Lipotor Lescol Pravochol		✓ ✓ ✓ ✓ ✓	✓ ✓ ✓ ✓ ✓
Antihypertension Drugs (Beta Blockers) (Ace Inhibitors) Zasotec			✓
K-Y Jelly	✓		
Fosomax (Bisphosphonates) (Also Actonel)		✓	
Evista (SERM)		✓	
ASA			✓
Bellergal			
Clonidine			
Lofexidene			
Megace			
Birth Control Pills		✓	

ALTERNATIVES FOR SYMPTOM RELIEF, PHYSICAL CHANGES, AND DISEASE PREVENTION			
Lifestyles	**Symptoms: Hot Flashes**	**Vaginal Dryness**	**Mood Swings**
Exercise Aerobic			✓
Weight Training			
Yoga			✓
Dress in Layers	✓		
Habits: Avoid Alcohol Avoid Caffeine Cessation of Smoking	✓ ✓	✓ ✓	
Diet: Animal Protein Plant Protein High Fiber Phytoestrogens (See listing part V, chapter 34)	✓		✓

ALTERNATIVES FOR SYMPTOM RELIEF, PHYSICAL CHANGES, AND DISEASE PREVENTION			
Lifestyles	**Sexual Dysfunction**	**Prevention**	
		Osteo	**CVD**
Exercise Aerobic	✓		✓
Weight Training		✓	
Yoga		✓	
Dress in Layers			
Habits: Avoid Alcohol Avoid Caffeine Cessation of Smoking		✓ ✓ ✓	✓
Diet: Animal Protein Plant Protein High Fiber Phytoestrogens (See listing part V, chapter 34)		✓ ✓ Not Studied	✓ ✓ Not Studied

Chapter 28

A First Look at Alternatives to HRT

Herbals and vitamins have emotional appeal, but they haven't been rigorously studied scientifically. They are not Food and Drug Administration (FDA) controlled, and the benefits listed on the packaging are derived mostly from reports of clinical usage and anecdotes. You should look these up in the resources listed to get details regarding dosage and adverse effects. Information about herbals is available in the resources listed following part V of this workbook and in the appendix to this chapter. The additional information in the appendix comes from some investigative studies of herbals reviewed and collated by the German "E" Commission, the European equivalent of our FDA. A good way to use this chapter is to locate, by symptom relief, those herbals you are interested in and then look them up below or in the resources recommended in part V.

Now that you have completed part IV, go to part IV of the MAP and fill it out, reflecting your work here.

HERBALS				
Name	**Source**	**Form/Dosage**	**Notes**	**Contra-Indications**
Bioflavionoids	Inner peel of citrus fruits, greens, bourbon	Capsules/250 mg 5-6 times daily	A diuretic; take with Vitamin C	None known
Black cohosh, Black snakeroot, bugbane, squawroot, cimicifuga racemosa	Plant of buttercup family	*Tincture: 10-15 drops daily; powder: 150-500 g daily; pills: 2 tabs twice daily (20 mg each)	For incontinence, 10-60 drops in a cup of tea daily; acts in the body like estrogen	Headaches, dizziness, nausea, visual disturbances; avoid if bleeding heavily, do not exceed 6 months
Calcium (fumarate, malate citrate succinate, aspartate, carbonate forms only)	Mineral found in milk, calcium carbonate, calcium citrate (best)	Premenopause: 600-1000 mg daily, menopause and postmenopause: 1200-1500 daily	Requires magnesium, B6 & D for absorption	Absorption is decreased by diets high in fiber, protein, caffeine & salt plus phosphates (sodas)
Chamomile Tea	Plant (flower)	Dried for tea tincture 3 times daily		
Chickweed, Stellaria media	Plant	Tincture 25-40 drops 1-2 times/day	Takes 1-2 weeks to work	
Dandelion, Taraxacum oficiniale, Pu gong ying	Garden Weed	Capsules: 1000-3000 mg daily; Tea leaf: 2-3 cups daily; Tincture: 2 tsp 3 times daily		A diuretic: too much may cause dehydration
*Tinctures are the most effective methods of taking herbs; made by soaking the herb in alcohol; dispensed in stopper bottles.				

HERBALS (CONTINUED)				
Name	**Source**	**Form/Dosage**	**Notes**	**Contra-Indications**
Dang qui, Dong quai, Angelica sinensis	Plant	Tincture: 10-40 drops 1-3 times daily; Dried root for tea: 4 to 8 oz. daily	Enhances E; Not a plant estrogen	Causes skin sun sensitivity; avoid if fibroids, bloating, diarrhea, or blood thinning durgs present
Elderflower, Sambucus	Plant	Tincture: 25-30 drops 2-3 times daily	Sets body's thermostat; get results in several days	
Flaxseed, Linum Usitatissimum	Plant	Oil: 1-3 tsps in AM Seeds: grind on food or soak in PM and drink in AM	Store oil in refrigerator; benefit ceases if discontinued	Cramping
Garden Sage, Salvia Officinalis	Plant	Tincture: 15-40 drops 1-3 times daily; Dry Leaf: 1-2 tsps in tea 8 times daily	Use as spice in cooking or drink as tea; acts in body like estrogen and progesterone	High doses harm kidney and liver; avoid if breast cancer present, can cause seizures
Gingko biloba	Extract from tree	Pills: 80 mg 3 times daily (up to 480 mg daily)	Aids memory, improves blood flow to brain, use of brain glucose, transmission of nerve messages	Headaches, GI upset; cannot take with aspirin, causes hemorrhaging

HERBALS (CONTINUED)				
Name	**Source**	**Form/Dosage**	**Notes**	**Contra-Indications**
Ginseng (Siberian & Korean) Eleutherococcus Senticosus	Plant	Tincture: 5-40 drops hourly; 500 mg capsules 1-3x daily	Aids memory, mental abilities; enhanced with E or flaxseed	Side effects; jitters, postmeno bleeding, high blood pressure, insomnia, skin eruptions, diarrhea; do not take with Vitamin C
Hops, Humulus, Lupulus	Plant			
Ipriflavone	Plant pigment flavored	Pill: 200 mg 3x daily with calcium	May halt bone loss	
Lady's mantle, Alchemilla vulgaris	Plant	Tincture: 5-10 drops 3 times daily; up to 2 wk/m	Take 1-2 weeks before period	
Licorice, Glycrrhiza globra	Plant: No relation to candy	Fluid: 1 tsp; Solid 250-500 mg; Powder for tea: 1-2 gm	Helps adrenal hormones make body produce estrogen from stored fat	Do not take if hypertension or heart problems present
Magnesium	Mineral found in nuts, seeds, whole grains, vegetables, chocolate	Pills: often combined with calcium, up to 450 mg daily (gluconate or citrate)	Third most prevalent mineral in bone	Diarrhea; deficiency results in no bone building and calcium deposit in soft tissue
Melatonin	Hormone available as a supplement	Pills: 3-10 mg 2 daily	Doesn't cause a hangover	Some pills have harmful impurities

HERBALS (CONTINUED)				
Name	**Source**	**Form/Dosage**	**Notes**	**Contra-Indications**
Mexican Wild Yam, Dioscorea villosa	Plant		Close to bodily estrogen; source of chemical used to produce first contraceptive	
Motherwort, Leonurus Cardioca	Plant	See each use Tincture: 20 drops 3 times daily		Do not use with other heart meds; avoid if heavy menstrual bleed or if at risk for breast cancer
Phosphorus	Mineral found in red meat, sodas; supplements not needed	Ratio of phosphorus to calcium should be 1.5 to 1	Second most prevelant mineral in bone	Excess causes bone loss
Red Clover, Trifolium Praetense	Plant	One tbsp. in tea daily		
Saint John's Wort, Hypericum Perforatum	Plant	300-500 mg tabs Tincture 3x daily		Takes 4-8 wks to take effect
Soybeans/ Soy products	Plant Beans, tofu, miso soy milk	Avoid pills 50-100 mg isoflavones daily	Active ingredients genestein and daizedin	

HERBALS & VITAMINS				
Name	**Source**	**Form/Dosage**	**Notes**	**Contra-Indications**
Valerian, Valeriana officinalis	Plant	Tincture: 20-30 drops at bedtime		Can be habit-forming
Violent, Viola	Plant	Dried leaves in tea; 1 cup daily		
Vitamin A	Meat, fish, eggs, carrots, spinach, canteloupe melon	5000 to 25000 IU beta-carotene with 5-15 mg zinc	Found as precursor, beta-carotene; needs zinc to convert it to usable form	High doses can yellow skin
Vitamin B6, Pyridoxine	Bananas, beans, fresh water fish, poultry	Pills: 50 mg twice daily	A coenzyme in production of progesterone; helps breast tenderness	B vitamins should be taken together to get better absorption
Vitamin C, Ascorbic acid	Citrus fruits	Pills: 1-2 g daily		
Vitamin D	Produced by skin under sunlight	Pills: 300-400 IU daily	Required for absorption of calcium	Deficiency leads to rickets
Vitamin E	Aloe	Caps: 1 g daily	Also good for dry skin; a building block to estrogen	Tends to interfere with treatment of breast cancer; excess interferes with blood clotting

HERBALS & VITAMINS				
Name	**Source**	**Form/Dosage**	**Notes**	**Contra-Indications**
Vitamin K	Synthesized by colon bacteria	No supplement required	Necessary for bone building and blood clotting	Deficiency can result from prolonged use of antibiotics
Vitex, Chaste tree; Angus castii (chaste berry)	Plant	Tincture: 20 drops twice daily; Caps: 3 daily; Tea: 1 cup/day; All = 30-40 mg	Shrinks fibroids Relieves PMS with 6-13 month regular use	None known
Wild yam root	Plant	400 mg/oz topical creams plus gels	All prescribed hormones except Premarin are **synthesized** from this plant	
Zinc	Cod, Turkey, Kidney beans	Pill: 15-30 mg/day	Sold bound to other minerals	

Part V

Alternatives

Chapter 29

What is Meant by "Alternatives"?

Women ask me frequently, "What can I do for myself?" By now, you've gotten my message that menopause is universal; we can live 40 percent of our lives in the postmenopause years; and, viewed positively, menopause can be the starting point for healthy change.

We rely a great deal on prescription medications for treating symptoms and disease. I think this is because we're not taught how to evaluate change of life symptoms (some are time-limited, some aren't, and most are not indicators of future health problems). Also, modern medicine is slanted toward treating illnesses after they have occurred, while more and more of us are seeking professional advice about prevention and wellness. This means that we'll have to take part of the responsibility for our health by addressing lifestyle changes we'll need to make. This is hard to do, and a little scary, because we don't have specific answers to the question, "Is what I'm doing now going to protect me from getting sick later?" Instead, we're used to medicine doing the work for us.

I was in the lady's lounge in one of my favorite restaurants (in the stall, actually) when I overheard this conversation between a mother and her daughter.

"Now, tell me again, how much of the bread, potatoes, and ice cream do you think you had?" said the mother.

Her daughter replied, "I can add another unit of insulin to this dose now, and maybe more later."

They were trying to calculate how much more medication would be needed to compensate for all the extra starches and sugars the diabetic daughter had eaten. They were planning to use the medication to try to keep her from becoming hyperglycemic and sick due to overeating. See what I mean: their focus was on suppressing symptoms with medication; it wasn't on self-regulation, advance planning for eating out, and making better food choices.

Menopause is not a chronic and potentially debilitating disease like diabetes. Most women do not require specific medical management for menopause. But all women require maintaining a healthy lifestyle and most women need to make lifestyle changes.

QUIZ

Answer the following questions:

How's your health right now? Circle your answer:

Excellent   Good   Fair   Poor

Are you being treated for any medical problems? Circle your answer: Yes   No

If your answer was "Yes," list these problems:

_____

_____

_____

Is your current treatment working? Circle your answer: Yes   No

If your answer was "No," have you been advised to make some lifestyle changes? Circle your answer: Yes   No

Are you experiencing hormone-related symptoms (peri-menopausal, menopausal, or postmenopausal symptoms)? Circle your answer: Yes   No

If your answer was "Yes," list them and grade them (1) mild, (2) moderate, or (3) severe.

Symptom   Rating

_____   _____

_____   _____

_____   _____

_____   _____

_____   _____

_____   _____

Which lifestyle changes have you made in the last year?

_____ Weight loss

_____ Smoking cessation

_____ Vitamin and mineral supplementation

_____ Physical activity (exercise)

_____ Prescription therapies

_____ Nonprescription therapies

_____ Stress management therapies

Which ones are you considering making in the coming year?

_____

_____

_____

Please write a brief explanation of why you want to make these lifestyle changes: _____

_____

How much time can you devote to your lifestyle changes…
    Daily?   _____
    Weekly?   _____
    Monthly?   _____
    Quarterly? _____
    Yearly?   _____

Complementary and alternative medicines (CAMs) are often referred to as "natural therapies." Treatment with these therapies is based on influencing the body's recuperative functions and preventing disease. Many CAM treatments have not been investigated or proven effective by rigorous scientific study, and much of what we know about how they work is based on observation. What we do know is that many of these therapies have been used for thousands of years.

Many of us are already using alternative treatments for our menopausal symptoms. In 1997, the North American Menopause Society (NAMS) conducted a survey that reported that 80 percent of their respondents were using such treatments as diet, vitamin and mineral supplements, herbals, yoga, and lifestyle changes rather than prescription medications. There is the general perception that CAM therapies focus on the body as a whole and emphasize wellness rather than illness.

There is no one treatment that can be used for all women in treating menopause symptoms. But the goals of these therapies apply to all women: to optimize health during and after menopause.

CIRCLE YOUR ANSWERS

Are you getting an annual physical exam?   Yes   No

Are you getting treatment for psychological problems?
   Yes   No

Are you getting treatment for acute perimenopause symptoms?
   Yes   No

Are you getting counseling for potential chronic disease?
   Yes   No

The most important functions of CAM therapies sought by women are to provide symptom relief, to aid in hormone output in the body, and to prevent disease in the postmenopausal years.

In 1992, the National Institutes of Health (NIH) established an Office of Alternative Medicine, which was renamed in 1998 as the National Center for Complementary and Alternative Medicine.

There are more than three hundred types of CAM therapies. The National Center for Complementary and Alternative Medicine has classified CAM therapies into categories. The following are therapies most commonly used by women to treat their menopausal symptoms:

- *Mind-Body Medicine.* Mind-body medicine involves behavioral and spiritual approaches to health. Examples include yoga, hypnosis, and meditation.
- *Alternative Medical Systems.* Examples include acupuncture, Oriental medicine, naturopathy, and homeopathy.
- *Lifestyle Change and Disease Prevention.* These are accomplished through general nutritional intervention and naturopathy.
- *Biologically Based Therapies.* Examples include herbs, vitamins, and minerals.

• *Manipulative and Body-Based Systems.* Examples include chiropractic medicine and massage.

Quiz

Have you been using any of these CAM therapies? What might your reasons be for choosing CAM therapies (check all that apply)?

_____ Dissatisfaction with prescription medicine.

_____ Concerns about HRT side effects and long-term effects.

_____ To gain more personal control over your own health.

CAM therapies, as an "ideal" alternative to HRT, would have the following properties:

• Prevent heart disease
• Prevent osteoporosis
• Protect the uterus and breasts from cancer
• Relieve the symptoms of menopause without restarting the menstrual cycle (the most common reason women stop taking HRT)
• Produce no side effects such as those experienced with prescription medications (the second most common reason women stop taking HRT)

We know these therapies are highly effective for symptom relief. Intensive research, however, is going on to assess their ability to enhance hormone output and prevent future disease.

Women are using nontraditional medical approaches to treat their symptoms. These alternative medical systems are not taught in medical school or covered by insurance plans. It is beyond the scope of this chapter to explain them in detail but, briefly, these include:

Naturopathy

Naturopathy blends centuries-old nontoxic therapies with current health advances and is considered a class of effective menopause therapies. It is primary health care performed by a doctor of naturopathy who has completed four years of graduate training in natural therapies applied to family health care. Write down the name, address, and phone number of a naturopathic physician in your area:

Homeopathy

Homeopathy describes illnesses as physiologic imbalances that can be corrected. It focuses on plant-derived remedies in small doses to combat symptoms and address imbalances associated with menopause. Write down the name, address, and phone number of a homeopathic health-care provider or pharmacist in your area:

Acupuncture

Acupuncture is a component of Chinese medical care dating back more than twenty-five hundred years. Acupuncture involves stimulation of anatomical locations on the skin. It is used for pain relief, prevention of illness, and performance enhancement. In the field of psychiatry, acupuncture is effective for the treatment of depression, anxiety, insomnia, pain, alcoholism, and drug and tobacco abuse. Write down the name, address, and phone number of a practitioner in your area:

Biofeedback

Biofeedback techniques have been used to control hot flashes and reduce the frequency of incontinence. Write down the name, address, and phone number of a PhD-level psychologist practicing these techniques in your area:

_____

Later chapters will focus on the forces of good: nutrition, herbal medicines, and exercise; but first, the forces of evil: tobacco and alcohol.

Chapter 30

Smoking

Why do we do it?
Quiz

If you smoke, answer the following questions:

When did you start? _____

Who first introduced you to cigarettes? _____

Do you smoke throughout the day? _____

Do you smoke primarily during certain activities? _____

If your answer was "Yes," what activities are they? _____

_____

Check all that apply:

_____ You smoke to control your nerves.

_____ You smoke to reduce weight.

_____ You smoke to calm frustration.

_____ You smoke to relieve boredom.

_____ You smoke to decrease anxiety in social situations.

Check all that apply:

_____ You smoke a lot at home.

_____ You smoke a lot in the car.

_____ You smoke a lot at work.

_____ You smoke a lot with friends.

How much do you smoke in a week?_____
How much do you spend on cigarettes weekly?_____

If you're smoking, you know you should stop, but I never responded to fear tactics and threats, and neither will you. So, here are some benefits from becoming a nonsmoker:

- Your kids will think well of you. Smoking is time-consuming. When I smoked, I spent a lot of time lighting up instead of playing with my kids.
- You can really reduce your risks for future disease, such as heart attack and cancer. Women who smoke have a four times greater chance of dying from a heart attack than women who don't smoke. *Lung cancer is strongly associated with smoking.* Overall, 35 percent of smokers will die of heart disease or lung cancer. If you stop smoking, in ten years your risk of heart disease and cancer diminishes to the same level as for nonsmokers.
- Bone loss is much less rapid and the risk of hip fracture is reduced. In the postmenopause years, women have a tendency to lose bone calcium, and our risks of getting osteoporosis increase with age.
- Dental health improves. For some women, estrogen depletion affects their gums and teeth, and smoking increases the risk of infection and tooth loss.
- You can delay the skin changes that are the early signs of aging. Smoking causes early skin wrinkling; the typical smokers' wrinkles are deep smile lines around the eyes and mouth. Smoking damages the small blood vessels in the skin, damages skin collagen, and delays skin healing. A forty-year old

woman who smokes can age her skin by twenty years! (This isn't a fear tactic, it's an appeal to your vanity...)

QUIZ

Are you considering quitting? Circle your answer: Yes   No

Write down the date you intend to quit:_____

Do you need help? Circle your answer: Yes   No

If your answer was "Yes," check your preferences:

_____ Medication

_____ Biofeedback

_____ Hypnosis

_____ Group therapy

Tips on How to Quit

Prepare to quit. Get out a sheet of paper. List all of the reasons why you want to quit smoking. Write down your previous practice sessions (times you tried to quit) and what made you go back to smoking. Identify the times, places, activities, and people that trigger you to smoke. Think of ways to deal with those and write them down.

Choose the date you will quit. Pick a date and stick to it. Choose a date that will give you enough time to prepare. Pick a date that may be special, such as an anniversary, a holiday, the Great American Smokeout, etc. Write the date down and place it somewhere so that you can see it every day.

Learn about recovery (withdrawal) symptoms and how to cope with them. Have your support person or system ready to go. You may (or may not) experience recovery (withdrawal) symptoms such as:

- Feeling irritable
- Having cravings
- Having headaches or feeling dizzy
- Having a dry mouth
- Having insomnia and/or vivid dreams
- Having an upset stomach
- Coughing
- Feeling fatigued
- Having difficulty concentrating
- Feeling restless

Help yourself recover: drink plenty of water, walk, exercise (see your doctor first), relax, eat low-calorie snacks, and avoid caffeine.

Don't be discouraged by relapse. If you smoke a cigarette and still want to quit, try again. Everyone has practice sessions. Smoking is one of the hardest behaviors you will ever have to give up. You can do it. Be prepared and remember the benefits: quitting will make you a happier and healthier person.

And ladies, quit after your period. Withdrawal symptoms are aggravated by PMS. Check with your doctor about an appropriate level of exercise for you, and exercise regularly while quitting. Exercise relieves the symptoms of withdrawal. Unless you are overeating or drinking, weight gain after quitting is usually five to seven pounds. If you exercise while quitting, you can actually lose weight.

Chapter 31

Alcohol, Soda, and Caffeine

Men and women differ a lot when it comes to handling alcohol. I noticed this when I was in college and graduate school (my heavy drinking years). We weigh less, we have less stomach enzyme to break down alcohol before it gets into the bloodstream, and we have more body fat. Therefore, when men and women drink the same amount of alcohol, it breaks down more slowly so more of it is circulating in our bloodstream, and it gets concentrated in our body fat. Those organs that are damaged by high concentrations of alcohol are the liver, brain, and breast tissue. Men metabolize alcohol more quickly and pass it more quickly.

Here's a quiz to test your general knowledge about alcohol.

QUIZ

True or False — Circle your answer.

T F Moderate alcohol consumption at bedtime can help you sleep. F: studies have shown that bedtime alcohol consumption causes insomnia and, even worse, it can trigger hot flashes and night sweats.

T F Drinking can make you look older. T: even moderate drinking affects the skin and hair; it worsens acne and dandruff through dehydration of your cells and dilation of tiny blood vessels in the face and nose; and it causes collagen and elastin damage, causing brown spots.

T F Moderate amounts of alcohol are good for you. F: even though there's still controversy over the health benefits of alcohol, most studies indicate that alcohol has no real nutritional value; furthermore, alcohol contains seven calories per gram, as compared to four calories per gram of protein and carbohydrate and nine calories per gram of fat. Since metabolic rate declines during perimenopause, most of these calories are stored as fat; weight gain is common in drinkers. Heavy drinkers have low bone mass because they have poor diets often deficient in calcium and vitamin D; moreover, alcohol interferes with calcium and vitamin D absorption into the bone tissue—this combination increases the risk of osteoporosis.

T F Drinking can increase your breast-cancer risk. T: perimenopausal women who drink are increasing their risk of breast cancer by 11 percent if they have one drink per day, by 24 percent if they have two drinks per day, and by 38 percent if they have three drinks per day; it is speculated that alcohol causes damage to the DNA in breast cells and interferes with your immune system's ability to resist infection and destroy precancerous cells.

T F Excess drinking is getting drunk. F: excess, for women, means more than two drinks a day.

T F Alcohol enhances sexual feelings. F: alcohol can both lower inhibitions and increase promiscuity (thereby increasing the risk of contracting sexually transmitted disease) while suppressing orgasms.

How much is too much? One drink is defined as twelve ounces of beer, five ounces of wine, or one and one-half ounces of liquor (these contain 5 percent, 10 percent, and 40 percent alcohol, respectively). Moderate drinking is not more than one drink a day. Heavy drinking is two drinks a day. More than this is excessive.

How do you know if you have a serious problem with alcohol? To determine whether you might be abusing alcohol, answer and score the following questions:

Quiz

_____ Tolerance — How many drinks does it take to make you feel high? If the answer is more than two drinks, score yourself 2 points.

_____ Annoyed — Have people annoyed you by criticizing your drinking? Score 1 for yes.

_____ Cut down — Have you felt you ought to cut down on your drinking? Score 1 for yes.

_____ Eye opener — Have you ever had a drink first thing in the morning to steady your nerves or get rid of a hangover? Score 1 for yes.

_____ Total — If the total of the scores for your answers to these questions is 2 or more, you may be abusing alcohol.

Alcohol consumption can be habit forming, so be careful not to let it sneak up on you. Consider the following and circle your answers.

Do you come from a family of heavy drinkers?　　　Y　　N

Do any of your close relatives have a drinking
　problem?　　　　　　　　　　　　　　　　　　Y　　N

Do you use diet pills, painkillers, or tranquilizers?   Y   N
If you drink, did you start as a teenager
   (or younger)?   Y   N
Do you skip meals when you drink?   Y   N
When you drink, do you eat a lot of high-fat foods? Y   N

These are some of the factors that can increase your chances for abusing alcohol.

Here are some tips to help you drink safely and to help protect you from alcohol's toxic effects.

- Limit yourself to one drink a day or less.
- Drink beer, or dilute wine and spirits in other beverages.
- Alternate alcoholic with nonalcoholic beverages.
- Be aware that alcohol stimulates your appetite for fatty foods.
- When you drink alcohol, drink two to three glasses of other fluids afterward.
- If you don't drink, don't start; there are better ways to enjoy yourself without relying on alcohol.

The Food and Drug Administration reports that excessive intake of alcohol, soda, and caffeine are the major causes of malnutrition in adult Americans.

- Are you drinking more than ten ounces of soda daily?
- Are you drinking more than three cups of caffeinated coffee daily?
- Are you at risk for thinning bones?

Both caffeine and phosphates in soda are suspected of increasing dehydration and calcium loss from bones. Even mild dehydration will slow down your metabolism as much as 3 percent, and almost 2 percent of Americans are chronically dehydrated. Dehydration is the number one trigger of daytime fatigue. Calcium loss puts you at risk for osteopenia and osteoporosis.

Finally, some sodas have unadvertised (but not unpublicized) benefits. Cruising the Internet, I found, for example,

- To clean a toilet, pour a can of Coca-Cola into the toilet bowl and let it sit for one hour, then flush clean; the citric acid in Coke removes stains from vitreous china.
- To clean corrosion from car battery terminals, pour a can of Coca-Cola over the terminals to bubble away corrosion.
- To loosen a rusted bolt, apply a cloth soaked in Coca-Cola to the rusted bolt for several minutes.
- The distributors of Coke have been using it to clean the engines of their trucks for about twenty years!

Whether the above is credible or not, there is a growing suspicion among nutrition research scientists that excessive soda consumption is partly responsible for the increased prevalence of gastrointestinal disorders (gastric reflux problems) and osteopenia (low bone density) in middle-aged women.

Try this experiment. Take a six-week break from drinking any carbonated beverage. What do you notice?

First, can you stop your soda intake for this long? Sugar and caffeine together in soda make a powerful addictive stimulant and, if you're having trouble temporarily eliminating soda, you are probably hooked on the habit of drinking it.

Have you switched from regular to diet sodas to lose or avoid gaining weight? You're probably not getting the weight loss you thought you would. The colorings and flavorings in sodas are sugar-based, and you're not completely eliminating sugar with diet varieties. If you have diabetes, you'll need to eliminate soda completely from your diet.

Have you noticed more belching, burping, mild gastric pain, and indigestion when drinking soda, particularly with a meal? Soda can overstimulate gastric acid production and, in some of us, aggravate gastric conditions.

Does soda satisfy your thirst? Drinking soda usually increases the thirst sensation, encouraging you to drink more of it. Soda also increases hunger, so that you consume snacks (mostly carbohydrates) while drinking it.

Here's my point: soda isn't really nutritious, but it does have a place in a food plan. Instead of consuming it as a dietary staple, drink it as a treat, infrequently and in small quantities.

Chapter 32

Vitamin and Mineral Supplements

If you've never really taken supplements before, why do you need them now?

This chapter is about nutrition. The science of nutrition is about an underlying belief in the body's ability to heal itself and prevent disease, and the emphasis of nutrition is on influencing these processes. Many midlife women are nutritionally impaired, meaning that our bodies have lost much of their ability to heal, protect against, and prevent disease.

QUIZ

Are you one of the 50 percent of women between the ages of forty-five and sixty who have one or more of the following health problems? Circle all that apply.

- Obesity
- Hypertension
- Diabetes
- Thyroid disease
- High cholesterol
- Low bone density
- Heart disease

Good nutrition is important at any age, but crucial at midlife because we're losing the protective effects of estrogen and because all the years of accumulated bad habits are slowly but surely catching up to us.

Quiz

Which of these is important to you? Rank them in order of importance, 1 to 6. I want to improve my nutrition:

_____ To support and protect my health for the last half of my life, even though I've always taken my health for granted.

_____ To minimize emerging health problems and/or stabilize current health problems.

_____ To control and eliminate weight gain.

_____ To boost my overall hormone output from all my glands (pituitary, thyroid, adrenals, and ovaries).

_____ To lessen menopause symptoms.

_____ To delay the appearance of aging.

The human body requires forty-five or more vitamins and minerals to maintain health. Researchers from the United States and Canada working with the Institute of Medicine and the National Academy of Sciences have established the recommended dietary allowance (RDA) of these nutrients. Vitamins and minerals are substances that your body requires to help regulate metabolic functions within cells and only very tiny amounts of them are required, usually less than one gram a day for the entire body.

The following is a sample list of vitamins and some of their functions. In general,

- Vitamins A, E, and K help repair cells in organ tissues;
- Vitamin B-complex is used by the nervous system;
- Vitamin C helps in the repair of blood vessels;
- Vitamin D with calcium and magnesium is involved in bone and muscle health and in the regulation of our body water.

Is it true or false that you can meet most of your daily requirements by eating properly?

False: here are some examples of the quantity of food it would take to get the recommended daily requirement of some common vitamins/minerals:

- 1,500 mg of calcium daily is equal to one quart of low-fat milk, one quart of low-fat yogurt, or ten cups of cottage cheese;
- 2,000 mg of vitamin C is equal to twenty-eight oranges;
- 30 IU of vitamin E is equal to three ounces of wheat germ;
- 5,000 IU of vitamin A is equal to seven mangos.

Now, no one eats twenty-eight oranges a day. And yes, there are other foods containing vitamin C, which could be eaten daily, along with that orange. You could have grapefruit and a salad with tomatoes and peppers along with lunch, and broccoli and potatoes along with dinner with strawberries for dessert. Almost every food has nutrients in it if it hasn't been overly processed or filled up with additives or overcooked. Where will you get your food from, and how will it be prepared? You will probably have to eat a lot of food and consume a lot of calories (and spend a lot of money) to get what you need.

There are two things to remember about vitamins:
- Our bodies absorb and use vitamins in food better than those in vitamin supplements.
- Vitamin-rich food increases the absorption of the supplement so that less of it becomes a waste product in the bowel or urine.

Without overeating, the best and easiest way to get these nutrients is with supplements, and the best way to take these supplements is with vitamin-rich food.

I was asked recently what I thought of the specially packed supplements advertised as the *High Energy Complexes*, which are usually specific vitamin combinations with a limited number of vitamins (such as B-complex only). My experience with these is that I don't absorb them well and my urine turns bright yellow as they are, for the most part, eliminated. It makes more sense to me to take multivitamin formulations since vitamins and minerals actually need each other for absorption and utilization. Therefore, I think your multivitamin supplement is a better "high energy" supplement than a supplement that's limited in vitamin and mineral content.

How nutritious is your diet? Use the Diet Log that follows to record your food and drink intake for a week. Following the Diet Log is a chart of essential nutrients and their sources. Check the nutrient if you eat or drink one or more of its source foods daily. Are you eating your way into good health daily?

DIET LOG

MEAL	Sunday	Monday	Tuesday	Wednesday
Breakfast				
Lunch				
Dinner				
Bedtime Snack				

Nutritional Supplement
Multivitamin____Calcium____
Antioxidants____Other_____
Protein Supplement:_____
Midmorning____Afternoon____Evening____

DIET LOG

MEAL	Thursday	Friday	Saturday
Breakfast			
Lunch			
Dinner			
Bedtime Snack			

Nutritional Supplement
Multivitamin____Calcium____
Antioxidants____Other_____
Protein Supplement:_____
Midmorning____Afternoon____Evening____

NUTRIENTS AND THEIR SOURCES

<u>Nutrient</u>	<u>Sources</u>	<u>**Eat Daily**</u>
Vitamin A	Orange and yellow fruits, vegetables, liver, egg yolks, fortified milk	_____
Or Beta-carotene (vitamin A precursor)	Orange and yellow fruits, vegetables	_____
Vitamin D	Fortified milk, sardines, sunlight	_____
Vitamin E	Whole grains, nuts, vegetable oils	_____
Vitamin C	Citrus fruits, broccoli, green and red peppers, brussels sprouts, tomatoes, strawberries, cabbage, potatoes	_____
Folic Acid	Green leafy vegetables, enriched cereals, legumes	_____
Thiamine	Whole and enriched grains, beans, pork	_____
Riboflavin	Milk, cheese, eggs, green leafy vegetables, whole and enriched grains	_____
Niacin	Meats, poultry, fish, whole and enriched grains	_____
Vitamin B6	Green leafy vegetables, meats, poultry, fish	_____
Vitamin B12	Meats, fish, milk, eggs, yogurt	_____
Calcium	Milk, cheese, yogurt, tofu, sardines, green vegetables	_____
Selenium	Water, shellfish, nuts, legumes	_____
Iron	Meats, fish, poultry, legumes, whole and enriched grains	_____
Zinc	Meats, whole grains, legumes, nuts	_____
Chromium	Whole grains	_____
Essential Fatty Acids (Omega-3 Fatty Acids)	Fish, fish oils, flaxseed, canola oil	_____

It may be helpful to be even more specific. If grains are a good source of iron, what grains are particularly high in iron? If fish are a good source of essential fatty acids, which fish are particularly good? Here's a list of food groupings and those foods in each grouping that are particularly high in nutrients.

Plant

Grains—whole wheat, brown rice, buckwheat, millet, cornmeal, oatmeal, whole grain pastas

Beans—navy, black, adzuki, chickpeas, lentils, kidney, pinto, soy

Vegetables—(above and below ground) dark leafy greens, asparagus, potatoes, yams, mushrooms, napa cabbage, bok choy, cabbage, beets, garlic, butternut squash, artichokes, seaweed

Fruits—berries, citrus, figs, black currants, avocados, apples, plantains, apricots

Nuts and seeds—almonds, walnuts, chestnuts, hazelnuts, cashews; sunflower, sesame, pumpkin seeds

Animal

Fish—salmon, mackerel, herring, tuna, trout, oysters, shrimp, clams

Meats and poultry—chicken, beef, lamb, game, organic liver, pork

Dairy

Milk, cheese, yogurt

Other

Fats and oils—extra virgin olive oil, flaxseed oil, unrefined sesame oil, unsalted butter

Whole grains top the list because they are full of fiber, vitamins, minerals, and other nutrients. If you have an allergy to wheat (which is more common that you think), you'll need to avoid whole grains but, from the listing, there are plenty of other highly nutritious foods that can replace these. If you're not already eating some of these foods, I encourage you to incorporate them into your diet.

Quiz

What three foods do you eat all the time?

_____

What are your three favorite foods?

_____

What groups are these from?

_____

Pick from the food list at least three substitutes you would like to try.

_____

Variety will help you get the nutrients you need and make your diet interesting.

Recent studies from across the United States and around the world have focused on the antioxidant properties of certain vitamins, particularly vitamins C, E, and beta-carotene (the precursor of vitamin A). Antioxidants destroy certain molecules in the body called free radicals, which are known to contribute to many diseases, including heart disease and many types of cancer. Does this mean we should take megadoses of vitamins? No. You risk an overdose, or waste your money on a measure that may or may not prove to be successful in the long run. *You should try to get your vitamins and minerals first from foods (without overeating) and second from supplements, and remain within the guidelines set forth by the U.S. Food and Drug Administration.*

The following is a list of supplements recommended for midlife women by many researchers and clinicians working in the field. Do you take supplements? If so, list their quantities on the appropriate lines. How do your supplements measure up? They should provide the minimum recommendations. Circle the deficiencies. Do they add up to three or more? If so, you need to consider changing your supplements and/or adding to them. If you don't take supplements, you should consider it.

SAFE LIMITS FOR VITAMINS AND MINERALS

Vitamins	Daily Value	Upper Level	Your Supplement
Vitamin A	5,000 IU	10,000 IU	_____ *
Vitamin B1 (thiamine)	1.5 mg	None Set	_____ *
Vitamin B2 (riboflavin)	1.7 mg	None Set	_____ *
Vitamin B3 (niacin)	20 mg	35 mg	_____ *
Vitamin B6 (pyridoxine)	2 mg	100 mg	_____ *
Vitamin B12	6 mcg	300 mcg	_____ *
Folate (folic acid)	400 mcg	1,000 mcg	_____ *
Vitamin C	2,000 mg	10,000 mg	_____ *
Vitamin D	400 IU	2,000 IU	_____ *
Vitamin E (natural only, "d" form)	30 IU	800 IU	_____ *
Vitamin K	80 mcg	80 mcg	_____

Minerals	Daily Value	Upper Level	Your Supplement
Calcium	1,500 mg	2,500 mg	_____ *
Chromium	120 mcg	400 mcg	_____ *
Copper	2 mg	10 mg	_____
Iron	18 mg	45 mg (only if deficient)	_____
Magnesium	750 mg	1,200 mg	_____ *

(The RDA ratio for women of calcium to magnesium is 2 to 1)

Phosphorus	1,000 mg	4,000 mg	_____
Potassium	1,800 mg	6,000 mg	_____
Selenium	70 mcg	400 mcg	_____
Zinc	15 mg	40 mg	_____ *

Other	Daily Value	Upper Level	Your Supplement
Boron (needs calcium for absorption)	3 mg	20 mg	_____
Iodine	150 mcg	1,100 mcg	_____
Manganese	2 mg	11 mg	_____
Molybdenum	75 mcg	2,000 mcg	_____
Nickel	5 mcg	1,000 mcg	_____
Vanadium	10 mcg	1,800 mcg	_____
Essential Fatty Acids (Omega 3, 6, 9 from fish, beans, soy, or plant oils)	7 mg weekly	None Set	_____

It is very important that the starred (*) nutrients not be deficient.

You'll notice that some of my vitamin ranges are higher than the product you're currently using. Should you increase specific vitamin amounts by adding to them? No. Don't supplement your supplement with more pills. These supplements are not a substitute for eating nutritious foods. Use food to boost your vitamin intake. In this way, you won't run the risk of exceeding the recommended daily limits, you'll have better absorption of your supplement, you won't inadvertently starve your body of necessary nutrients, and you will eat well.

In order to take supplements safely, you should be able to answer "yes" to the following questions.

- Are you taking a multivitamin rather than megadoses of single vitamins?
- Are you taking your vitamins with food rather than as a substitute for a meal?
- Does the meal contain some fat to aid in absorption?
- Have you checked the expiration date on your bottle to make sure your vitamins are still potent?
- Do you buy your supplements from a national brand or major chain store to assure quality? The letters "USP," for United States Pharmacopoeia, are a sign of quality.
- Have you checked with your doctor about possible good and bad interactions with medications you are taking?
- Is your diet well-rounded (meaning you eat a variety of foods) and your first source of vitamins and minerals?
- And, for the safety of your pocketbook, are you spending more than 20 cents a day for supplements? Paying more doesn't mean better quality.

In case you're not familiar with product labeling practices, here's a diagram on how to read a supplement label.

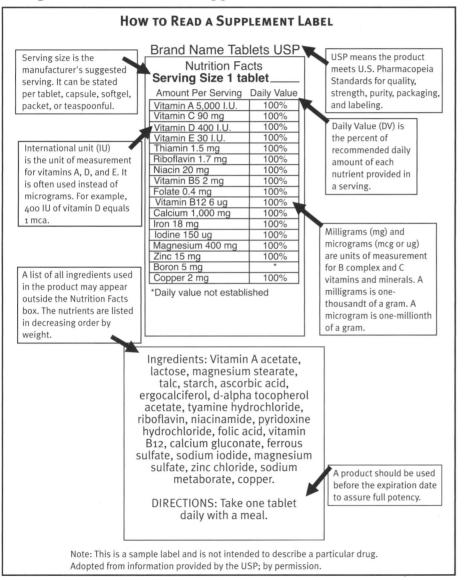

HOW TO READ A SUPPLEMENT LABEL

Brand Name Tablets USP

Serving size is the manufacturer's suggested serving. It can be stated per tablet, capsule, softgel, packet, or teaspoonful.

USP means the product meets U.S. Pharmacopeia Standards for quality, strength, purity, packaging, and labeling.

International unit (IU) is the unit of measurement for vitamins A, D, and E. It is often used instead of micrograms. For example, 400 IU of vitamin D equals 1 mca.

Daily Value (DV) is the percent of recommended daily amount of each nutrient provided in a serving.

A list of all ingredients used in the product may appear outside the Nutrition Facts box. The nutrients are listed in decreasing order by weight.

Milligrams (mg) and micrograms (mcg or ug) are units of measurement for B complex and C vitamins and minerals. A milligrams is one-thousandt of a gram. A microgram is one-millionth of a gram.

Nutrition Facts
Serving Size 1 tablet_____

Amount Per Serving	Daily Value
Vitamin A 5,000 I.U.	100%
Vitamin C 90 mg	100%
Vitamin D 400 I.U.	100%
Vitamin E 30 I.U.	100%
Thiamin 1.5 mg	100%
Riboflavin 1.7 mg	100%
Niacin 20 mg	100%
Vitamin B5 2 mg	100%
Folate 0.4 mg	100%
Vitamin B12 6 ug	100%
Calcium 1,000 mg	100%
Iron 18 mg	100%
Iodine 150 ug	100%
Magnesium 400 mg	100%
Zinc 15 mg	100%
Boron 5 mg	*
Copper 2 mg	100%

*Daily value not established

Ingredients: Vitamin A acetate, lactose, magnesium stearate, talc, starch, ascorbic acid, ergocalciferol, d-alpha tocopherol acetate, tyamine hydrochloride, riboflavin, niacinamide, pyridoxine hydrochloride, folic acid, vitamin B12, calcium gluconate, ferrous sulfate, sodium iodide, magnesium sulfate, zinc chloride, sodium metaborate, copper.

DIRECTIONS: Take one tablet daily with a meal.

A product should be used before the expiration date to assure full potency.

Note: This is a sample label and is not intended to describe a particular drug.
Adopted from information provided by the USP; by permission.

What You Need to Know, Nutrient by Nutrient

Vitamin A (or beta-carotene) may be taken in doses of 5,000 IU daily. Vitamins A, C, and E are antioxidants. They bind up oxygen-free radicals and keep them from causing the kind of damage that speeds up the aging process in all the cells of the body. The best sources of vitamin A in plants are carrots, sweet potatoes, spinach, and cantaloupe; in animals, beef liver, fish, and fish liver oil. Vitamin A is essential for bone growth and repair, healthy skin, and night vision. It's fat-soluble (can only be absorbed in the presence of fat) and, in large doses, can be toxic. ALERT: overdose can cause fetal malformations in pregnant women, and liver damage. A 1996 study suggested that very large doses can worsen heart disease and lung cancer. Newer studies indicate that the current recommended daily value may be too high, and that 2,500 IU is a safer guideline.

Vitamin C (Ascorbic Acid) can be taken in doses of 2,000 mg daily in divided doses. Most of this is excreted in the urine three to four hours after having been taken, so ingesting several doses through the day is optimal. Sources are most fruits and vegetables, particularly orange juice, kiwi fruit, broccoli, and raw tomatoes. Well-researched, it has been proven that vitamin C reduces LDL (bad) cholesterol in heart disease; increases collagen formation in the skin and prevents skin aging; assists the absorption of dietary calcium from the intestine for use by the bones; prevents some toxic effects of alcohol (it helps avoid hangovers); inhibits the formation of cancer-promoting free radicals taken in when eating foods such as hot dogs, bacon, and processed meats; reduces the risk of death from all cancers by 14 percent by influencing the immune system to respond to the cancer cells; prevents cataracts; helps absorb dietary iron from the intestines; and plays a role in the formation of adrenaline, our stress reaction hormone. It enhances the effectiveness of echinacea in fighting infection. ALERT: fever; high stress; smoking; and taking aspirin, antibiotics, and steroids all deplete the body's stores of vitamin C. In these situations, take more vitamin C (up to 10,000 mg daily; excess will be eliminated in the stool). The signal that you are taking more than you need is loose stools.

Vitamin E (d-alpha tocopherol) may be taken in doses of 400 to 800 IU daily. If you are taking large doses, split them up throughout the day; vitamin E is best absorbed in increments of 400 IU or less. It is fat-soluble and should be taken with food containing fat. Its absorption is helped by the presence of selenium (a mineral). Sources are bran, wheat, nuts, seeds, fish, crab, vegetable oils, and sweet potatoes. Vitamin A and beta-carotene can reduce blood levels of vitamin E, so increase your intake of E if you are taking more than 5,000 IU of vitamin A daily. Vitamin E has a blood-thinning effect; caution is advised when taking it with anticoagulants and aspirin. It is contraindicated if you are being treated for breast cancer or diabetes because it can interfere with absorption of medication. Vitamin E is useful orally and topically for treating dry skin, orally for treating hot flashes, and via internal application for vaginal dryness. An antioxidant like vitamins A and C, it helps prevent cell damage and plays a positive role in the prevention of stroke and death in coronary artery disease. ALERT: avoid synthetic vitamin E. Natural vitamin E is produced from vegetable oils, mostly soybean oil; synthetic vitamin E is produced from petrochemicals. Recent studies confirm that synthetic vitamin E is useless. This is how to tell the difference between them: natural vitamin E is labeled as "d-alpha tocopherol"; synthetic vitamin E is labeled as "dl-alpha tocopherol." Be careful. Overdose can be toxic.

The B-Complex is made up of vitamin B1 (thiamine), B2 (riboflavin), B3 (niacin), B6 (pyridoxine), and B12 (folate, or folic acid). They are all water-soluble, and they all help convert carbohydrates into glucose for immediate energy. Midlife women use B vitamins to relieve PMS symptoms and dryness of skin and hair.

Vitamin B6 is particularly important for midlife women. It prevents coronary heart disease and helps form serotonin, which helps decrease PMS symptoms. It is also useful in treating insomnia and irritability in depressed women. ALERT: large doses (more than 200 mg daily) should be avoided because of the possibility of occurrence of abnormal neurological symptoms.

Vitamin B12 is needed to make red blood cells. A deficiency causes pernicious anemia, a common condition in older adults because of lower production of stomach acid to help absorb this vitamin from food. Sources are all animal foods. Supplements are well absorbed in older adults.

Folate (folic acid) is needed in the formation of red blood cells. It reduces the risk of heart attacks, and it helps in the prevention of colon cancer. Sources are green leafy vegetables and oranges. Some foods have been fortified with a folic acid supplement, but it needs the other B vitamins for absorption.

Vitamin D may be taken in doses of 400 IU daily. Sources are canned tuna and salmon, fish liver oils, whole milk, butter, beef liver, egg yolk, and exposure to the sun for fifteen minutes daily (ultraviolet rays convert cholesterol molecules in the skin to vitamin D). Note: dietary vitamin D must have vitamin A present for absorption in the intestine. Vitamin D helps absorption of dietary calcium by the bones, reduces the risk for colon cancer, and, research indicates, may help prevent breast cancer. Without vitamin D, absorption of dietary calcium is impaired and the risk of osteoporosis goes up.

Calcium (calcium citrate) may be taken in doses of 1,000 to 1,500 mg daily. As a matter of interest, this is the equivalent of five eight-ounce glasses of milk. Our bones are not inert objects, but living tissue that receives and releases calcium daily. Calcium is necessary for bone density and, after menopause, it is estimated that women lose 5 percent of their bone density every year. Calcium deficiency is hard to detect because calcium levels in the blood may appear normal: when the body needs calcium for normal muscular functioning, bone strength, blood clotting, and nervous system integrity, it will "steal" calcium from teeth and bones to raise low blood levels. Only 10 to 20 percent of calcium found in foods is actually utilized. Supplements can be taken with and without meals so long as other nutrients are present for absorption. To be absorbed, calcium needs an acid environment in the stomach, vitamins A and D, amino acids (such as leucine, arginine, and serine), magnesium, and phosphorus. Our bodies prefer calcium supplements in small doses of 500 mg, taken with a multivitamin to aid absorption. ALERT: calcium carbonate has the highest calcium content of any supplement but is an antacid; calcium needs stomach acid to be absorbed and, as we age, we produce less stomach acid. For the older adult, calcium supplements made from calcium citrate offer better absorption. Calcium absorption is decreased in diets high in alcohol, caffeine, fruit, fiber, protein, and salt, or low in vitamin D. Calcium is useful for the replacement of bone mineral mass and has a mild sedative effect when taken at night. A frequent problem with taking calcium supplements is constipation. The National Academy of Sciences and the National Institutes of Health recommend the following daily intake by age:

- Age 19–30: 1,000 mg
- Age 31–50: 1,000 mg
- Age 51–65: 1,200 mg
- Age 65 and older: 1,500 mg

Magnesium may be taken in doses of 500 to 750 mg daily. Sources are wheat bran, nuts, seeds, fish, milk, grains, and green vegetables. Magnesium's functions are similar to those of calcium in the body, and it is needed to absorb dietary calcium. For optimal effectiveness, take a dose of magnesium equal to half the dose of your calcium citrate supplement. ALERT: excesses of protein, dark green leafy vegetables, and alcohol deplete magnesium. Magnesium plays a role in the prevention of hypertension and osteoporosis. It maintains the heartbeat (low levels lead to arrhythmias), and it reduces the buildup of fatty deposits in the blood vessels. Magnesium also provides relief from migraine headaches. Diuretics, antibiotics, and alcohol decrease its absorption. Diabetes contributes to magnesium deficiency. Signs of deficiency are heartbeat irregularities, muscle weakness, dizziness, and tremors. Chronic deficiency may lead to increased risk of diabetes.

Potassium may be taken in doses of 1,800 to 6,000 mg daily. It is found in most foods but is especially concentrated in apricots, avocados, bananas, brown rice, dried fruit, garlic, nuts, wheat bran, and yams. Potassium maintains a regular heartbeat and stabilizes blood pressure by controlling the body's water balance and sodium content, and by assisting in proper muscle contraction. ALERT: stress, diuretics, and laxatives deplete potassium levels in the body.

Chromium helps insulin regulate blood sugar. Sources are grains and mushrooms. Chromium picolinate is a heavy metal taken for weight loss. At 200 to 400 mcg daily, it can increase the burning of calories and induce weight loss, but its safety is in question, even at recommended doses.

Iron may be taken in doses of 10 to 18 mg daily only if you have been proven to be iron-deficient. All cells in the body contain iron. It is an especially crucial element in hemoglobin, the oxygen-carrying protein that gives blood its red color, and in certain muscle tissue. However, recent studies indicate that many Americans may be suffering from iron overdoses. Scientists believe that iron may well act as an oxidant in the blood, promoting a reaction between LDLs and oxygen that results in atherosclerosis and coronary artery disease. This means that unless you are suffering from excessive abnormal bleeding, you should not take iron supplements. ALERT: women have fewer heart attacks before menopause because they maintain relatively low iron stores during the menstrual years. Women do lose iron every month with their menstrual period, but most seem to get enough iron in their food to forestall anemia. When the menstrual periods stop, iron levels rise in post-menopause and so does heart attack risk. All the iron we need is supplied in our diets; don't supplement unless you are iron deficient.

Zinc may be taken in doses of 15 to 30 mg daily. It is a trace element found in many foods. Sources particularly high in zinc are pumpkin seeds, oysters, herbs (especially sage), and Mexican wild yam. Zinc is needed for the functioning of the immune system. ALERT: large doses (more than 2,000 mg daily) are toxic.

Omega-3 Fatty Acids are not vitamins or minerals, but polyunsaturated fats. I've included them with vitamins and minerals because they are essential. This supplement lowers the risk for coronary heart disease. The best source is fish: the fatter the fish, the higher their omega-3 fatty acid content. The American Heart Association recommends getting 7 grams of omega-3 fatty acids per week; as little as four servings of fish every week can significantly lower a woman's risk for heart disease. Here's what you'll get in a four-ounce cooked serving of different types of fish:

Type of Fish	Grams of Omega-3s
Herring	2.4 g
Pacific Mackerel	2.1 g
Atlantic Salmon	2.1 g
Sablefish	2.0 g
Whitefish	1.9 g
Pink Salmon (canned)	1.9 g
Atlantic Sturgeon	1.5 g
Tuna (albacore)	1.5 g
Red (sockeye) Salmon	1.4 g
Bluefish	1.2 g
Eastern Oysters	1.0 g
Whiting (hake)	1.0 g
Bass (freshwater)	0.9 g
Swordfish	0.9 g
Tuna (white, canned)	0.8 g
Sardines (canned)	0.7 g

Other sources of Omega-3 fatty acids include flaxseed oil, soybeans, and canola oil.

Food & Fitness Advisor, June 2002, Volume 5, Number 11.

What You Need to Know about Foods, Drugs, and Metabolic Conditions That Deplete Vitamin and Mineral Levels

Protein—If you eat more protein than required for nutritional purposes, it is not stored by the body, but must be excreted. Excess protein waste products are excreted in the urine. The excretion of protein waste products through the kidneys increases the urinary excretion of calcium. A high intake of protein creates a negative calcium balance (more is lost than ingested). A negative calcium balance will cause calcium to be pulled from the bones and teeth.

Diuretics—Some diuretics cause increased urinary excretion of minerals such as calcium and potassium. Furosemide (Lasix) promotes the greatest loss of calcium. Others, such as thiazides, do not promote such loss.

Antibiotics—Broad-spectrum antibiotics kill friendly intestinal bacteria that make vitamin K for us. Vitamin K is a bone-building factor. Long-term or frequent courses of antibiotics result in low vitamin K levels and thereby interfere with bone building. If antibiotics must be used long-term or frequently, it is wise to supplement vitamin K and replenish friendly colon bacteria such as L. acidophilus. Take both as long as you are taking antibiotics, and for two to four weeks afterward.

Flouride—A potent enzyme inhibitor, fluoride causes pathological changes in bone, leading to increased risk of fracture. Fluoride in all forms, including toothpaste, should be avoided by everyone. Fluoridation is associated with increased incidence of hip fractures. Humans can tolerate a low level of fluoride in their drinking water, but it is now generally acknowledged by scientists that the supposed dental benefits of higher fluoride levels to children's teeth have been false, as fostered by early fluoride studies.

Cortisone—People placed on long-term use of large doses of glucocorticoids will develop osteoporosis. These medications are prednisolone, triamcinolone, methylprednisolone, and dexamethasone.

Anticoagulants—If you are taking blood thinners, you should not take large amounts of vitamins A, E, and K because they increase the blood-thinning effect, which can result in excessive bleeding.

Metabolic Acidosis (as in fad diets)—One of the body's responses to high acidity is to buffer the excess acid with calcium, usually taken from bone for the purpose. This weakens the bones.

Hyperthyroidism—accelerates bone loss and thus promotes osteoporosis.

Well, that's it on supplements. On to food itself.

Chapter 33

Food Basics:
Protein, Carbs, Fats, Fiber, and Water

This is what you need to know about carbs, fats, proteins, fiber (a type of carbohydrate), and water—the basics of food.

Carbohydrates circulate through the bloodstream in the form of glucose and are our primary energy source. Excess is stored as glycogen in the liver or converted to fat and deposited in fat cells around the body.

There are three types of carbohydrates: simple sugars and refined carbohydrates; complex carbohydrates; and fiber.

The *simple sugars* are honey and fruits. *Refined carbohydrates* are, for example, white flour, refined sugar, and white rice. Sugar is a great source of instant energy because it doesn't need to be digested to be absorbed. However, it is low in vitamins and contains no fiber, so has little nutritional value. High blood sugar causes high amounts of insulin to circulate in the bloodstream, and insulin converts sugar into fat and stores it. The result? Obesity.

Complex carbohydrates are so called because they need to be digested to be absorbed. These are chiefly starches such as potatoes, corn, beans, and vegetables. They are high in nutritional value. Vegetables, grains, and fruits are full of fiber, which is the indigestible portion of these foods, as well as vitamins and minerals.

Fiber is actually a complex carbohydrate found in most vegetables and fruits. There are two kinds: insoluble, which increases bulk in stool, for example, whole grains; and soluble, which traps and removes cholesterol from the intestine, for example, vegetables, beans, and fruit. The recommended allowance is 30 to 40 grams daily. ALERT: high fiber can cause constipation, gas, and bloating. Add it to your diet gradually.

Quiz

What kind of carbohydrates do you eat?

_____

Are most of your carbohydrates simple or complex?

_____

List three complex carbohydrates.

_____

What high fiber carbohydrates do you eat? List two.

_____

"Above ground" vegetables have a lot of vitamins and minerals; which do you eat? List three.

_____

Do you eat beans and whole grains? Circle one:
    Daily   Weekly   Monthly
Do you eat potatoes/pasta/white rice? Circle one:
    Daily   Weekly   Monthly

Most Recommended	*Least Recommended*
Grains and beans	Sugar, flour, white rice
"Above ground" vegetables	"Below ground" vegetables
Fresh fruit	Peeled or canned fruit

Fats (also called lipids) make up a large category of compounds. The dietary fats are saturated fats, hydrogenated fats, polyunsaturated fats, and monounsaturated fats, as well as cholesterol, triglycerides, and omega fatty acids.

Fats are overrepresented in the American diet. Are they solely the cause of our high rates of cardiovascular disease? We used to think so, but there's mounting evidence that excessive amounts of carbohydrates and fats together are the culprits. We don't yet know enough about fat metabolism. Several research questions are currently under rigorous study. Are saturated fats truly a dietary enemy? Does dietary fat consumption alone affect blood cholesterol levels? Does it do so directly or indirectly? How much dietary fat is too much?

This is what we do know.

Fat is actually one component of a broad category of substances called lipids. Lipids include fats, fatty acids, sterols, and other compounds that are not soluble in water. Although not all lipids are fats, the terms are often used interchangeably. Cholesterol, for instance, is categorized as fat when, actually, it is a lipid. We do need fat to provide our bodies with essential fatty acids, which are the raw material for several body functions, including proper cell growth and blood pressure control.

There are several kinds of dietary fat, each with its own distinctive properties.

Saturated fats are found in animal foods and dairy products. Most of these fats are solid at room temperature. Examples are butter, cheese, lard, and chocolate.

Hydrogenated fats are the fats in oils, processed foods, margarine, and shortenings.

Polyunsaturated fats are liquid at room temperature. Examples are vegetable oils such as corn and soybean oil.

Monounsaturated fats are found in olive oil, peanut oil, and canola oil, and these are helpful because they reduce the tendency for cholesterol to be deposited in the arteries.

Fish oils are beneficial because they lower triglyceride levels and help blood clotting. Omega-3 fatty acids are found in high concentration in sardines, salmon, tuna, mackerel, and herring. Note: fish oil capsules can raise LDL cholesterol levels; it is best to get fish oil by eating fish once or twice a week.

Triglycerides are found in most fatty foods. For women, high levels of this fatty acid put them at high risk for coronary heart disease.

Cholesterol is a lipid (waxy substance) found in animal foods and dairy products. Cholesterol is vital to our existence: it builds cell membranes and it is the basic building block for hormones. The body can manufacture all the cholesterol it needs; it's not necessary for us to ingest it, yet the average American consumes anywhere from 600 to 1,500 mg of cholesterol every day. It comes in two forms; low-density lipoproteins (LDLs), which carry lipids into the bloodstream, and high-density lipoproteins (HDLs), which tend to carry lipids out. Cholesterol is found in a wide variety of foods.

Quiz

Which categories of fat make up most of your dietary fat?
    List them. _____

How often do you use vegetable oils in preparing your meals?
    Circle one.   Daily   Weekly   Monthly

Where does most of your cholesterol come from? Circle one.

Animal foods   Dairy products

Do you eat fish? Circle one.   Daily   Weekly   Monthly

Do you have any of the following? Check all that apply.

_____ Obesity

_____ Hypertension

_____ High cholesterol

_____ Diabetes

Are you under a doctor's care? Circle one.   Yes   No

Are you on a diet? Circle one.   Yes   No

Is your diet helping you

_____ Lose weight?

_____ Lower blood pressure?

_____ Lower cholesterol?

_____ Lower blood sugar?

Most of us believe that if we cut out our dietary fat, we will be healthier. Research is finding out that low fat consumption alone is not the remedy we used to think it was.

Protein forms the structure of all the parts of the body. Our bodies make protein by assembling amino acids into chains; eight essential amino acids cannot be manufactured by our bodies and must be supplied by the food we eat. Meat, fish, and poultry contain all eight essential amino acids; fruit and vegetables do not. Too much protein in your diet causes calcium loss and too little protein leads to malnutrition and, eventually, starvation. To maintain our supply of essential amino acids, we need daily protein, but not in large quantities. There are two sources of protein, animal and plant. The animal proteins require calcium for digestion and therefore cause a steady depletion of bone calcium over time, unless we get it in our diet. Plant proteins do not deplete bone calcium.

Quiz

What kinds of proteins do you eat predominantly, plant or animal? List a few. _____

How often do you eat protein? Circle one.

Daily   Weekly   Monthly

Do you eat red meat (a source of high-fat protein)? List three sources. _____

Do you eat fish or poultry (sources of low-fat protein)? List three sources. _____

Protein does not have to be high in fat content to be nutritious.

Do you use protein supplements?

_____

Does your protein supplement contain all the essential amino acids? (The label will tell you.) _____

Water is the most abundant substance in our bodies and every cell is flooded with it. You probably didn't know that dehydration will cause death much more quickly than starvation. We actually need more water as we age, and most of us don't drink enough of it. Besides the water in our food, we need eight additional eight-ounce glasses daily. Caffeinated and carbonated drinks all contain water, but they also leech calcium out of our bones. Caffeine is a diuretic (which is why coffee and tea seem to move right through you) and, of course, alcohol is also dehydrating.

Quiz

Circle Yes or No.

Do you get hunger pains less than two hours after eating?	Y	N
Do you snack when you're feeling irritable?	Y	N
Do you get sleepy during the middle of the afternoon?	Y	N
Do you start your day with coffee or tea?	Y	N
Does it take an hour or two to feel awake in the morning?	Y	N
Do you get tired too easily with just moderate exercise?	Y	N
Do you get frequent mild headaches during the day?	Y	N
Has it been hard to lose weight past a certain point?	Y	N
Do you feel bloated after meals and have gas pains?	Y	N
Are you constipated even though you get enough fiber?	Y	N
Are you drinking fewer than eight glasses of water a day?	Y	N

If you answered "Yes" to any of these questions you might be dehydrated. Liquids other than plain water ideally should be unsweetened (unflavored teas or coffees) or artificially sweetened, decaffeinated, and noncarbonated.

A more accurate calculation of the daily amount of water you need is this:

.04 x current weight in pounds x 2 = _____ cups per day.

How much water should you be ingesting? _____ cups per day.

Recommendations

Select unprocessed foods high in vitamins and minerals, i.e., fresh fruits and vegetables, not canned or prepared. Eat complex carbohydrates rather than simple or refined carbohydrates, i.e., fruits and vegetables, not sugar, white bread, white rice, or pasta. Eat more fruits and vegetables for their antioxidant content, too. Eat more fish, olive oil, and low-fat substitutes instead of red meat and whole milk dairy products. Increase your intake of fiber; eat lightly cooked fruits and vegetables and add beans (but be sure to drink plenty of water to avoid constipation). Nutritional supplements to consider are a multivitamin, calcium, and fiber. Antioxidant and protein supplements are optional. Eating from all the following food groups will give you variety as well as most of your vitamins and minerals. Most foods contain protein, carbohydrates, and some fat; the Xs in the chart show which are predominate in each food:

Plant	Protein	Fat	Carbohydrate
Grains	X		X
Beans	X		X
Above-ground vegetables	X		X
Below-ground vegetables	X		X
Fruits			X
Nuts and seeds	X	X	
Fats and oils		X	

Animal	Protein	Fat	Carbohydrate
Fish	X	X	
Meat and poultry	X	X	
Dairy	X	X	
Fats and oils		X	

Chapter 34

Phytoestrogens

Are you looking for alternatives to prescription medications for relief of your symptoms?

Are you unable to take prescription medications for your symptoms?

Do you think that nonprescription remedies are better for you than prescription remedies?

Have you heard of phytoestrogens?

Phytoestrogens are a large and varied group of plant-derived compounds that act like a weak form of estrogen in the body. There are many foods that contain phytoestrogens. Isoflavones are one class of phytoestrogens, lignans are another. The most well-known foods among isoflavones are soybeans and soy products, and the best-known herbs in this class are black cohosh and red clover. The best-known plant in the lignan class is flaxseed. Many women use isoflavones for relief of perimenopausal symptoms.

Here's a partial listing of these foods and herbs:

PHYTOESTROGEN-CONTAINING FOODS, HERBS, AND PLANTS

Alfalfa	Apples	Barley	Basil
Beans (red, green)	Black Cohosh	Buckwheat	Cabbage

Caraway	Cherries	Chervil	Chickpeas
Citrus Rinds	Clover	Corn	Dill
Flaxseed	Garlic	Ginko Biloba	Ginseng
Green Tea	Licorice	Oats	Parsley
Peas	Pomegranate	Primrose Oil	Red Clover
Red Sage	Rice Bran	Sarsparilla	Sesame Seeds
Soybeans	Soybean Shoots	Sprouts	Sunflower Seeds
Tofu	Wheat Bran	Wheat Germ	

These are all available at local markets and health food stores. Because there is such a wide variety of phytoestrogens, it is very easy to put them into your diet on a daily basis.

Many plant foods contain phytoestrogens, but none have as many estrogen benefits as soy. Soy is almost a "wonder food." It is one of the best sources of isoflavones; it contains high-quality protein (supplying most of the eight essential amino acids); and it is lactose-free, cholesterol-free, and a source of omega-3 fatty acids. And soy also contains calcium.

QUIZ

Phytoestrogens are reported to help alleviate the following perimenopause and postmenopause symptoms. Check the ones you are experiencing.

✓ Hot flashes	_____ Heavy bleeding
_____ Insomnia	✓ Irritability
✓ Mood swings	✓ Memory lapses
_____ Urinary incontinence	_____ Vaginal dryness
✓ Wrinkles	_____ Increased cholesterol levels

Are you taking phytoestrogens for these symptoms? What's your experience been? Are you getting symptom relief? Side effects? No results?_____

There has been some research conducted on soy. The recommended daily dose of soy isoflavones is the following: to reduce cholesterol, you will need about 20 grams of soy protein daily (the equivalent of 40 milligrams/day of isoflavones); to benefit bone health, you will need about 40 grams of soy (the equivalent of 80 milligrams/day of isoflavones); to relieve hot flashes, you will need 60 grams of soy (equivalent to 120 milligrams of isoflavones daily). These equivalencies are high. Moreover, as you might expect, some foods contain more isoflavones than others. Here is a list of foods and the average number of milligrams of isoflavones per 100 grams of that food.

ISOFLAVONE CONTENT OF FOODS

Food	Mg Isoflavones/100 g of Food
Soybeans, green, raw	151.17
Soy flour	148.61
Soy protein concentrate (water-washed)	102.07
Soy protein isolate	92.43
Miso soup, dry	60.39
Tempeh	43.52
Soybeans, sprouted, raw	40.71
Soybean curd (fermented)	39.00
Soy cheese, unspecified	31.32
Tofu (Mori-Nu), silken, firm	27.91
Tofu (Azumaya), extra firm, steamed	22.70
Tofu yogurt	16.30

Soy hot dog, unprepared	15.00
Soy protein concentrate (alcohol extraction)	12.47
Soy milk	9.65
Soy noodles, flat	8.50
Vegetable burgers, prepared (Green Giant, Harvest)	8.22
Soylinks, cooked (Morning Star Breakfast)	3.75
Frankfurters, canned, meatless	3.35
(Worthington, Loma Linda, Big Franks)	
Split peas, raw	2.42
Soy sauce (shoyu, made from soy and wheat)	1.64

Courtesy of the USDA–Iowa State University.

Whole foods are preferable to protein supplements as good sources of isoflavones. You can buy these products at natural food stores and specialty counters in some supermarkets.

Studies are going on right now to determine whether or not phytoestrogens can actually be used to treat menopause symptoms and protect against bone loss, heart disease, brain deterioration, and cancer. Soy products and red clover have been studied the most. Some results so far:

- On hot flashes and vaginal dryness—results similar to placebo, inadequate data so far
- On heart disease—whole soy foods daily seem to decrease total cholesterol and LDL (bad) cholesterol
- On bone loss—no findings, too few human studies
- On brain deterioration—no findings, too few human studies
- On cancer—soy has both protective and stimulatory effects on breast cancer, not enough research about uterine cancer or any other cancers

Phytoestrogen-Containing Herbs

There is no regulation of herbs and, thus, there's great variation in quality. Herbs can be taken in a number of forms: as a tea, an infusion, or as tinctures or fluid extracts. Tinctures are generally the most effective method of taking herbs. Pills are a grab bag: many are good, but others contain so little active herb that they're virtually worthless. If you're taking an herb in capsule form and it appears to be having no effect, consider trying a tincture or tea before abandoning it entirely. Stick to one herb, or wait until you have used one herb for a period of time before adding a second. Side effects from herbs are usually milder than those from drugs, but they do occur, as do allergic reactions. Most herbs are perfectly safe and the risk of toxicity is low, but never assume that if a little is good, more is better.

Chapter 28 has a listing of herbals and vitamins that are recommended for symptom treatment; please review it.

QUIZ

Circle Yes or No.

Is HRT contraindicated for your use?	Y	N
Has HRT been ineffective in giving you symptom relief?	Y	N
Has HRT given you unwanted side effects?	Y	N
Do you prefer to use nonprescription therapies for symptom treatment?	Y	N

If the answer to any question is "yes," you may want to consider using herbals. They are available in vitamin stores and at pharmacies specializing in compounding herbal remedies.

The terms phytoestrogens, phytochemicals, and isoflavones are all used interchangeably (and are sometimes confusing). Phytochemicals are all plant chemicals and include a subgroup known as phytoestrogens. Phytoestrogens have two subgroups: isoflavones and lignans. Isoflavones have been studied: the biologically active chemicals in these are daidzein and genistein.

When you are evaluating a soy product, for example, you want to know what its isoflavone content is per serving, since this is the biologically active part of the soy product. The higher the isoflavone content, the more likely it is to be beneficial in treating your symptoms.

For example, if you want to treat hot flashes, you will need to consume approximately 120 milligrams of isoflavones/day. Products whose isoflavone content/serving is spelled out on the label are the easiest to evaluate. Without such labeling, I'm afraid you'll have to carry with you the list of average isoflavone content per 100 grams of food, or just learn those numbers for the foods you prefer. Serving size is usually given in grams or ounces. For ease of doing math in your head while standing in the market, assume 4 ounces equals 100 milligrams. A product such as raw green soybeans may be labeled as containing 150 milligrams isoflavones per 100 grams (4 ounce) serving, so you know you'll have to consume 3 to 4 ounces (one serving) of this product daily to get the results you want. Similarly, if fermented soybean curd is labeled as containing 40 milligrams of isoflavones per 100 grams (4 ounce) serving, you'll know that you need to consume 12 ounces (three servings) of this product daily. You would have to drink 48 ounces of soy milk every day to reach isoflavone levels recommended as beneficial for hot flashes.

I don't recommend that you consume large quantities of soy products on a daily basis. I do recommend that you add some soy to your food plan as a staple along with green vegetables and fresh fruit.

Not all soy products are healthy. Even though more than 80 percent of vegetable cooking oil comes from soybeans, it has to be hydrogenated. This process produces trans-fatty acids in the cooking oil. These are the fatty acids that researchers have implicated in the development of coronary heart disease.

The FDA is planning to require the listing of trans-fatty acids on food nutrition labels. Currently, only saturated fat is listed and consumers have no way of knowing how much trans-fat is in a product. In the meantime, a new soybean has been developed that does not require extensive processing to convert it into oil, and it will be healthier to consume. It will be available in 2004.

Chapter 35

Weight Gain and Muscle Loss

Weight gain is usually an insidious problem that develops over time. We feel like we're getting older when, without changing any of our habits of the past twenty years, we put on weight. Some of us try dieting, which doesn't seem to work anymore. Some of us stop paying attention to eating: we eat what we want when we want and put off worrying about it. Suddenly, we realize that we're heavier than we've ever been in our lives. And, no matter what we try to do about it, we can't seem to get control over it. Do you have a weight problem? There's more than one kind. Refer to the BMI chart at the end of this chapter for normal weight ranges.

QUIZ
Circle Yes or No

Are you underweight (less than 19 on the BMI chart)?	Y	N
Do you fear getting fat?	Y	N
Are you frequently on a food-restrictive diet?	Y	N
Do you eat less than 1,200 calories a day?	Y	N
Do you "binge out" on certain foods?	Y	N
Do you exercise more than eight hours/week?	Y	N
Do you force yourself to throw up and/or use laxatives?	Y	N

If you have answered "yes" to three or more of these questions, you might have an eating disorder, which is a psychological problem that usually requires professional help.

If you're experiencing weight gain, is this the first time you've had a weight problem? If no:

At what age did you notice the problem? _____

Is there a family pattern of overweight/obesity?   Y   N

How old are you now?_____

Have you been struggling with losing weight?   Y   N

Using the BMI chart, find the row for your height in inches. Your ideal BMI ranges from 19 to 24. Your ideal weight range is between the weight corresponding to a BMI of 19 and the weight corresponding to a BMI of 24. If you are 66 inches tall, your ideal weight range is 118 pounds to 148 pounds. What is your ideal weight range? _____

What weight would you like to be? _____

Are your weight loss goals realistic compared to the weight ranges on the BMI chart? _____

We normally gain weight as we age. As an adult, what is the lowest you've ever weighed and how old were you?

_____

As an adult, what is the most you've ever weighed and how old were you? _____

What's the midpoint between these two extremes of weight?

_____

This is probably what most of us should weigh comfortably by middle age.

If the difference between your lowest adult weight and highest adult weight is more than fifty pounds, let's take a closer look at your habits to identify the causes.

Quiz

Circle Yes or No

Are you inactive?	Y	N
Do you smoke more than five cigarettes a day?	Y	N
Do you repeatedly start and stop diets?	Y	N
Are you taking three or more medications daily?	Y	N
Have you lost muscle definition in your arms and legs?	Y	N
Have you added fat on old and new areas on your body (back, arms, waist, hips, and thighs)	Y	N

Half of all women between the ages of thirty-five and fifty-five are overweight. What causes this problem? Here is a list of causes, those we can't influence and those we can. Check those that apply to you.

Quiz

_____ I am a woman. Because we are female, we store more fat than men. Sex makes a difference.

_____ Obesity runs in my family. Yes, there is a fat gene.

_____ I have body fat accumulating on my arms, back, and chest (in addition to my hips, buttocks, and abdomen). Body fat distribution is genetically determined.

_____ I have polycystic ovaries or hypothyroidism. These medical problems are known to cause weight gain and we suspect other problems, such as diabetes.

_____ I am at least forty years old and have been inactive for the last five to ten years. Muscle mass decreases with age and, with less muscle, we burn fewer calories.

_____ I overeat. For forty years, we have steadily increased the size of our food portions in the United States, so that most of us are eating too much.

_____ I prepare few fresh foods and eat mostly packaged, processed, or fast foods. Prepared foods have less nutrient value and, as we age, the rate at which we can absorb vitamins and minerals from our foods falls.

_____ I have reached menopause and am physically inactive. After menopause, loss of lean body mass accelerates. A particular weight gain of ten pounds may actually be a loss of five pounds of muscle and a gain of fifteen pounds of fat!

_____ I take antidepressants, antihistamines, beta-blockers, insulin, amaryl, glucatrol, glucovance, chemotherapy, steroids, lithium, tranquilizers, antipsychotic medications, or birth control pills. All of these are known to cause weight gain.

_____ I have more than one alcoholic drink per day. Alcohol gets metabolized as sugar and more than two drinks a day is considered excess for women.

_____ I smoke. In the short-term, smoking suppresses the appetite, but it eventually accelerates the loss of lean body mass.

The three most common causes of weight gain in women are use of medications, physical inactivity, and alcohol consumption. All three of these causes can be changed to eliminate weight gain.

How do you know if you have lost muscle mass? Here are a few simple tests.

- Stand straight and, without holding on to anything, bend one leg up and behind you; hold for a count of 5. Repeat, using the other leg.
- Stand up, without leaning against anything, and put on your slacks.
- Stand straight; rise on tiptoe slowly and hold for a count of 10 without holding on to anything.
- Lie flat on your back on the floor; get up to a standing position without using your hands.

Muscle strength is key to balance and coordination. When these falter, you've lost muscle mass and strength. Therefore, with the simplest activities, we can feel weakness and fatigue.

To set realistic weight-loss goals, refer to the BMI chart at the end of the chapter. Look down the left column until you find your height in inches. Then look across that row until you find your weight in pounds (A=_____). Move back along the same row until you find the weight of a healthy person your height whose BMI is 24 (B=_____). Move further back along the same row until you find the weight of a healthy person whose BMI is 19 (C=_____). Subtract the weight of a person whose BMI is 24 from your body weight (A-B=D_____). Subtract the weight of a person whose BMI is 19 from your weight (A-C=E_____). A realistic range of pounds for you to lose is from D to E.

Finally, when might you need medical management, i.e., medications and/or surgery, for obesity? If your BMI is at least 27 and you have elevated cholesterol and triglycerides, hypertension, atherosclerosis and heart disease, diabetes, arthritis, breast or uterine cancer, sleep apnea, or depression and anxiety, you need medical help. If your BMI is 30 or greater with no health problems, lifestyle changes alone will probably not be enough, and you will also need medical management.

The Body Mass Index Chart follows. A word of explanation of the activity levels referred to:

BODY MASS INDEX CHART

BMI	19	20	21	22	23	24	25	26	27	28	29	30	35	40
	HEALTHY						OVERWEIGHT					OBESE		
Height in Inches	Body Weight in pounds													
58	91	96	100	105	110	115	119	124	129	134	138	143	167	191
59	94	99	104	109	114	119	124	128	133	138	143	148	173	198
60	97	102	107	112	118	123	128	133	138	143	148	153	179	204
61	100	106	111	116	122	127	132	137	143	148	153	158	185	211
62	104	109	115	120	126	131	136	142	147	153	158	164	191	218
63	107	113	116	124	130	135	141	146	152	158	163	169	197	225
64	110	116	122	128	134	140	145	151	157	163	169	174	204	232
65	114	120	126	132	136	144	150	156	162	168	171	180	210	240
66	118	124	130	136	142	148	155	161	167	173	179	186	215	247
67	121	127	134	140	146	153	159	166	172	178	185	198	223	255
68	125	131	138	144	151	158	164	171	177	184	190	197	230	262
69	128	135	142	149	155	162	169	176	182	189	196	203	236	270
70	132	139	146	153	160	167	174	181	188	195	202	207	243	278
71	136	143	150	157	165	172	179	186	193	200	208	215	250	286
72	140	147	154	162	169	177	184	191	199	206	213	221	258	294
73	144	151	159	166	174	182	189	197	204	212	219	227	265	302
74	148	155	163	171	179	186	194	202	210	218	225	233	272	311
75	152	160	168	176	184	192	200	208	216	224	232	240	279	319
76	156	164	172	180	189	197	205	213	221	230	238	246	287	328

DAILY CALORIC NEEDS FOR WOMEN

General Activity Level	Daily Caloric Intake
Sedentary	Ideal Weight x 11
Moderately Active	Ideal Weight x 14
Active	Ideal Weight x 18

Sedentary means you have no scheduled physical activity; most of your physical activity is the result of working or performing household chores.

Moderately Active means you have a regularly scheduled program of aerobics/muscle strengthening performed at least four times/week (or two hours/week).

Active means you are an athlete and train for your sport daily.

Current Concepts and Practices

The body mass index (BMI) is now the standard for evaluating whether your weight is healthy for your height. I've included the BMI chart or you can use this formula to calculate your BMI:

Weight = A._____pounds

Height = B._____inches

BMI = [A divided by (B x B)] x 704.5 = _____

Sample calculation:

Weight = 160 pounds

Height = 66 inches

BMI = [160/(66 x 66)] x 704.5 = 25.88

If your BMI is lower than 19, you are underweight and might have muscle atrophy which can put you at serious risk for osteoporosis. If your BMI is 25 or more, you are overweight with an increased risk for developing diabetes, high blood pressure, high cholesterol, heart disease, and breast and colon cancer.

Research studies have shown that the configuration of your excess body fat is also important: an apple-shaped configuration (mostly fat around the waist) is associated with heart disease, and a pear-shaped configuration (mostly fat around the hips) is associated with breast and colon cancer.

The old USDA guideline for healthy weight ranges is flawed: it makes the assumption that weight gain is a normal process of aging and that older women should weigh more than younger women. The weight ranges are misleading: for the younger woman, these ranges correspond to a BMI between 19 and 25 (which is healthy to mildly overweight), but for older women, the BMI ranges between 21 and 27 (which may reflect reality but is not a guideline for health). Now we know that a sustained BMI of 25 or more for any woman is a risk factor for future disease.

There are medical guidelines for treating obesity. These are listed below. Please note that lifestyle changes are the cornerstone of any weight-loss program. If you have any of the diseases listed under *Comorbidities*, lifestyle changes alone will not be enough. There are prescription medications that can help, but without the prerequisite lifestyle changes, their effectiveness is minimal.

INTERVENTION BY BMI CATEGORY

BMI	Intervention
< 24.9	no treatment needed
25–26.9	lifestyle changes,* if comorbidities present
27–29.9	lifestyle changes plus drug therapy, if comorbidities present
30–35.1	lifestyle changes plus drug therapy
35–39.9	lifestyle changes plus drug therapy; surgery needed if comorbidities present
40	lifestyle changes, drug therapy, and surgery needed

*Lifestyle changes = diet, exercise, and behavior therapy

Bruck, L. "Weight Gain During Perimenopause: The Case for Early Intervention." *Menopause Management*, 1999; 8(6): 6-11.

Obesity is considered a causative factor for each of the following medical conditions (comorbidities):

- Elevated cholesterol and triglycerides
- Hypertension
- Atherosclerosis and heart disease
- Adult-onset diabetes
- Arthritis
- Breast and colon cancer
- Sleep apnea
- Depression and anxiety

Medications prescribed for obesity:

- Meridia, which makes one feel full.
- Xenical, which blocks absorption of dietary fat. Both are used long-term.

Many of us as physicians admonish you to lose weight, cut down on what you eat, and exercise, but fail to provide you with enough useful information on just how to do this. The next chapter is an effort to give you the information you need and teach you how to use it to lose excess weight and maintain a healthy weight.

Surveys indicate that 50 percent of women in the United States between the ages of thirty-five and fifty-five are overweight. The reasons for this are varied. We eat a lot of snack foods. We frequently diet so that our bodies become resistant to dieting. We use a lot of medications, many of which induce weight gain. We are low in muscle mass because of our inactivity. And our bodies are very efficient at storing excess fat (on the arms, back, buttocks, and thighs).

If you haven't developed cellulite before, this is the time in your life when you'll first notice it. Every woman develops it at some point in her life. It's a female phenomenon, and where it develops on your body is predetermined by your genes. Even thin women develop it. Its presence, however, is usually aggravated by being overweight.

What is cellulite? Anatomically, it's the superficial layer of fat just under the skin that encircles our bodies from the waist to the knees. This fat is held down under the skin as though it were trapped by a fishnet and it pushes up through the spaces in the netting, giving that telltale puckered appearance on the skin surface.

Don't be fooled by product hype. There is no cure for cellulite. But there are treatments that can improve the appearance of cellulite areas. The treatments are two-fold. One is to moisturize the skin and infuse the fatty layer below the skin with fluid. This can be done with skin creams and moisturizers, drinking plenty of water every day, and using treatments that massage the top layer of skin to bring more fluid into the fat tissue. The second is to reduce your body fat. Most women who have cellulite also have fatty excess. If you are overweight, you'll need to reduce your deep fat stores by exercise and dietary changes; some women prefer liposuction. If you are not overweight, you can improve the appearance of cellulite with exercises that target those areas of cellulite buildup; try resistance exercises for the hips, buttocks, and thighs. You can still have fats in your diet, but stick to poly- and monounsaturated foods. Avoid caffeine because it is a diuretic and you don't want to get dehydrated.

There are many treatments advertised for cellulite control. Many work, but the beneficial effects will disappear when you stop the treatments.

Cellulite isn't considered a medical problem, but weight gain is. A BMI of 25 or more is considered a medical problem. Obesity peaks for 50 percent of women during their fifties in Western societies, which is just around menopause. But gaining weight at menopause is not inevitable because many women don't.

How much weight gain is a problem? In postmenopausal women, if your BMI is consistently over 27, in three years' time you'll be at risk for hypertension, diabetes, and high cholesterol; after ten years, you could develop heart disease. We don't have enough studies yet on younger women, but there is some indication that in obese young women, estrogen conveys some measure of protection against developing these chronic diseases. However, after menopause, that protection could very well be lost. And remember: where your excess body fat accumulates is also important. Apple-shaped weight gain is associated with an increased risk of heart disease and pear-shaped weight gain is associated with an increased risk of breast and colon cancer.

Why are so many of us overweight, and what causes obesity?

I've made two lists of the factors we know about (reflected in the risk assessment for obesity you took earlier). There are factors we can't change and there are those we can.

Those factors we can't change are:

Sex — All women are more efficient than men at storing fat.

Family genetics — There is a fat gene; where on our bodies our fat is stored is also genetically determined.

Medical diagnosis — Thyroid conditions and polycystic ovaries are known to cause obesity; other medical conditions are being studied.

Age — Fat metabolism changes around menopause; we don't know what triggers this (maybe lowered estrogen plays a role).

According to a study conducted at the University of Maryland and published in the *2002 Fall Journal of Endocrinology and Metabolism*, these are the processes that change: lipolysis (the process whereby fat is released from fat cells for energy) is reduced by 75 percent, fat stores are maintained, and dietary fat uptake is increased so that fat storage expands; bone mass and muscle decrease with age (so we have less muscle to burn calories with); and our basal metabolic rate decreases with age, which means as we age we burn fewer calories in a resting state. The overall result for a middle-aged, inactive female is this: your ten-pound weight gain is probably an actual loss of five pounds of muscle and a gain of fifteen pounds of body fat.

Those factors we *can* change are:

Smoking—Many women smoke to suppress their appetite, but this becomes less and less efficient for weight control because it accelerates the loss of muscle mass; eventually, there is a lot less muscle to burn calories.

Poor diet—We eat too many foods of poor quality and, due to a decrease in our production of gastric acid as we age, we absorb fewer vitamins and minerals. The result is a deficiency in essential vitamins and minerals as we age, while at the same time ingesting empty calories which are stored as fat.

Medications—Many medications cause weight gain as a side effect; medication groupings which are known to cause weight gain are antidepressants and lithium, antihistamines, beta-blockers, steroids, chemotherapy drugs, diabetic medications, and some contraceptives. Check with your doctor to see if you're taking any of these and to see if substitutions can be made to less offending agents.

Alcohol consumption — Alcohol is a sugar and it gets metabolized as excess dietary sugar; too much alcohol (more than two drinks a day for women) causes vitamin and mineral deficiency and increased loss of muscle mass.

Overeating — Many studies indicate that over the past forty years, all of us in Western culture have increased our food portions to megasized meals.

Lack of exercise — Let's face it, many of us have had years of decreased physical activity prior to reaching menopause. Prior to my menopause, the last time I really ran hard and long was when playing college sports. As couch potatoes, we are at risk for rapid loss of muscle mass in our postmenopause years.

Do you have a weight problem? Are you at risk for obesity?

Use the Managing My Weight Daily Log on the next page for a few weeks. It will give you a closer look at your habits and behaviors, and it will help you identify the factors that could be contributing to your weight problem. And, after you've identified what your causative factors are, you can decide on strategies for change.

My point is this: obesity at any age is a serious problem, and weight gain is a serious problem at midlife. It is too easily ignored by women and their physicians as a natural consequence of aging. More usually, weight gain in healthy women in Westernized societies is due to poor diet, eating and drinking too much of the wrong things, and inactivity. Over time, an extra fifty calories a day (one chocolate chip cookie) can cause five pounds of weight gain in one year and fifty pounds of gain in ten years. So, don't ignore it and don't let your physician minimize it.

MANAGING MY WEIGHT DAILY LOG				
Date	Start (Current)	Monday	Tuesday	Wednesday
Weight (once weekly)				
Medications (list them) ———— ———— ————				
Habits: Exercise (list type) ———— ———— ———— Smoking Alcohol (# of drinks) **Food & Drink** Water (glasses per day) Soda/juices (oz. per day) Fast foods Cookies/cake/ snacks (high fat food) Fruits/vegetables **Appetite** Increased portion size Decreased portion size Ate more often (during day) Ate less often No change				

MANAGING MY WEIGHT DAILY LOG				
Date	**Thursday**	**Friday**	**Saturday**	**Sunday**
Weight (once weekly)				
Medications (list them) _____ _____ _____				
Habits: Exercise (list type) _____ _____ _____ Smoking Alcohol (# of drinks) **Food & Drink** Water (glasses per day) Soda/juices (oz. per day) Fast foods Cookies/cake/ snacks (high fat food) Fruits/vegetables **Appetite** Increased portion size Decreased portion size Ate more often (during day) Ate less often No change				

Another misconception is that after menopause our weight gain is permanent. It is true that after menopause our body metabolism slows down, our body fat gets redistributed to the abdomen, hips, and buttocks, and our fat tissue becomes a major source of estrogen production for us. But we can still lose weight. The fundamental things apply...we've got to burn more calories than we eat. At any age, controlled caloric intake and physical activity are necessary for women to lose weight and maintain a healthy body weight.

Chapter 36

Dieting and Exercise

Diet

Deciding what kind of diet is best for you is largely a matter of trial and error. What do you like to eat? List those foods you eat frequently and circle the ones you like most.

<u>Category A</u>	<u>Category B</u>	<u>Category C</u>	<u>Category D</u>
Meat, poultry, fish, dairy	Grains, pasta, rice	Below-ground vegetables	Above-ground vegetables
_____	_____	_____	_____
_____	_____	_____	_____
_____	_____	_____	_____
_____	_____	_____	_____
_____	_____	_____	_____
_____	_____	_____	_____
Rank:_____	Rank:_____	Rank:_____	Rank:_____

Rank each category: 1—eat very often
2—eat often
3—eat sometimes
4—eat rarely

Eating any kind of food, including fruits and vegetables, can cause you to gain weight if you consume more calories than you burn off. How many calories do you need a day? Refer to the BMI chart at the end of chapter 35. Find the most you could weigh for your height and still be described as healthy. If you are 5'6" tall, you can weigh as much as 148 pounds. If you are inactive, to reach and maintain this weight, you need to consume 11 calories/pound daily, or 11 x 148 = 1,628 calories daily. If you limit yourself to 1,628 calories daily, you will lose weight until you reach 148 pounds, and then you will plateau. If you are moderately active, you need 14 calories/pound daily, or 14 x 148 = 2,072 calories daily. If you limit yourself to 2,072 calories daily *and* get aerobic exercise three days a week, you will lose weight until you reach 148 pounds, and then you will plateau. So you can eat a little more and still lose weight if you exercise. The weight of 148 pounds is not an ideal weight, but a weight at which you can still be described as healthy. Plain talk, this means that at 5'6" with a medium build, you will have to live with being a size 12 instead of a size 10.

If you are overweight and just beginning an exercise program, the following chart may help you. It is suggested that you begin dieting at the lowest calorie level for the weight you wish to attain and increase your intake as your activity level increases. So, if you want to weigh 150 pounds, start your diet at 1,800 calories daily and go up to 1,950 calories daily if you get 30 minutes of aerobic exercise five days a week. This is a bit stricter than the formulation in the previous paragraph and may produce results a bit more quickly.

How many calories do you need a day?

If you are overweight and just beginning an exercise program, it is suggested you begin with the lowest calorie level for your weight. It is not recommended to go below 1,200 calories daily.

Activity Levels:
Beginning—No formal exercise routine (just starting out)
Low Activity—Aerobic exercise, 30 minutes 5 times weekly
Active—Aerobic exercise, 60 minutes 5 times weekly
Very Active—Aerobic exercise, 120 minutes 5 times weekly

Calorie Maintenance Levels				
Weight	**Beginning**	**Low Activity**	**Active**	**Very Active**
100	1200	1300	1400	1500
110	1320	1430	1540	1650
120	1440	1560	1680	1800
130	1560	1690	1820	1950
140	1680	1820	1960	2100
150	1800	1950	2100	2250
160	1920	2080	2240	2400
170	2040	2210	2380	2500
180	2160	2340	2500	2500
190	2280	2470	2500	2500
200	2400	2500	2500	2500
200+	2500	2500	2500	2500

Comparison of activity levels between the chart above and the BMI chart:

Calorie Maintenance Levels		**BMI Chart**
Beginning and Low Activity	equivalent to	Sedentary
Active	equivalent to	Moderately Active
Very Active	equivalent to	Active

It is not recommended that you consume fewer than 1,200 calories a day. If you are being treated for any medical condition, check with your doctor before starting any diet. If you are over forty, check with your doctor before starting an exercise program.

Eating is only a habit, and your focus should be on changing your eating habits for life. Since there is no single diet that is right for all women, here are six plans that work.

Pyramid Plans (USDA and Others)

You can access these plans on the USDA Food and Nutrition Information Center website: www.nal.usda.gov/fnic. These are good plans for those who:

- Refuse to eliminate any foods from their diets
- Believe all foods have a place in a healthy diet
- Pay attention to portion sizes (keep them small)
- Make exercise a priority

The USDA Pyramid emphasizes a diet in which 60 percent of all calories come from carbohydrates, 25 percent of all calories come from protein, and 15 percent of all calories come from fat. To convert this into grams per food group, multiply total daily calories by each percentage and then divide your results by 4 for carbohydrates and proteins, and by 9 for fats. If you're 5'6" tall and are getting aerobic exercise three times a week, following the

USDA guidelines you have a 1,700 calorie daily limit. On this diet, this means you should be consuming 1,020 calories from 255 grams of carbohydrates (multiply 1,700 by 60 percent, then divide by 4), 425 calories from 106 grams of protein, and 255 calories from 28 grams of fat daily.

Reducing fat intake will not produce weight loss. In fact, the most popular and successful diet plans involve manipulating carbohydrate intake.

Weight Watchers

This is a good plan for those who:
- Want the benefits of a pyramid plan
- Don't want to eliminate any foods
- Want to eat from all the food groups
- Prefer low-fat foods
- Enjoy peer activities and peer support

Macrobiotics

This is a good plan for those who:
- Are already vegetarians
- Do not eat meat or dairy
- Like organic vegetables and whole grains
- Avoid refined sugars
- Favor beans, lentils, and tofu

The Zone

This is a good plan for those who:
- Prefer a rigid division of calories among carbs, protein, and fat
- Don't need variety in their menu

- Choose to eliminate most saturated fats (meats)
- Choose to eliminate most refined carbohydrates (bread, pasta, rice)

Carbohydrate Addicts
This is a good plan for those who:
- Don't want to count calories
- Instead, will count the grams of carbohydrate in food
- Prefer high-protein, low-fat foods
- Can limit their fruit consumption

The Atkins Diet
This is a good plan for those who:
- Prefer to eat large quantities of animal fat (bacon, eggs, steak, cheese)
- Can severely limit fruit and vegetables
- Can give up pasta, bread, rice, and potatoes

Institute of Medicine
The IOM released new nutrition and exercise guidelines for healthy Americans in September 2002. These are flexible diets with approximately one hour/day of exercise. Everyone requires different amounts of exercise to prevent weight gain.

Now that you know something about these diets, are you interested in trying one of them? I deliberately did not mention my personal preferences because I want you to experiment with some of them until you find one that suits you. Remember, no single diet or eating plan is right for all women. Focus on changing your eating habits for life.

As we age, restricting calories alone becomes inefficient at achieving weight loss. So, I offer the following list of things to pay close attention to when dieting.

- Cut back on starches and sweets; we tend to store these calories as fat.
- Downsize your serving portions; avoid "megameals."
- Take vitamin supplements with vitamin-rich food for optimal absorption of these supplements.
- Protein is crucial if you are exercising (it's muscle food).
- Added fiber helps lower your cholesterol.
- Bone loss is our major problem, and we can't get enough calcium from food alone; take a supplement.
- Going completely fat-free isn't healthy; small amounts of dietary fats (unsaturated) and omega fatty acids are good for our hearts and blood vessels.
- Avoid dietary cholesterol; our bodies can make what we need and our cholesterol levels tend to rise after menopause.
- Reduce your consumption of processed foods, refined sugars, and flour; these put us at risk for diabetes.
- Drink up; we tend to become more easily dehydrated as we age—soda, coffee, and tea don't count. Drink water, too.
- Don't starve yourself back into the dress size you wore when you were twenty; instead, exercise. This will help you regain your shape.

Current Concepts and Practices

As we age, we must avoid obesity because it is the major risk factor in many of the diseases that postmenopausal women acquire (see chapters 13–22 for disease risks). Many women enter midlife with bone mass depletion, muscle loss, and increased body fat. It doesn't really matter whether you are slender or fat, you can still have these conditions and not know it because they are relatively silent until they begin to cause symptoms of medical illness.

Our diets are carbohydrate-rich and we are just beginning to understand that the quantity of carbohydrates as well as their quality are implicated in obesity. With aging, our bodies are less efficient at metabolizing carbohydrates, at absorbing vitamins and minerals from our food (for example, B12 and calcium), and using calories for energy. Our metabolism does get slower with age. Some researchers estimate that we'll need to subtract ten to fifty calories from our daily caloric requirement for each postmenopause year up to age seventy. We can reverse the trend to lower, slower metabolism with consistent exercise. And as long as we don't increase our food intake as we exercise, we can keep our metabolic rate up and maintain a healthy weight range.

Here's how to roughly calculate your basal metabolic rate (BMR), or the number of calories your body burns at rest:

Weight in pounds x 4.4	= _____	= A	For example, 160 x 4.4 = 704.0
Height in inches x 4.7	= _____	= B	66 x 4.7 = 310.2
A + B	= _____	= C	A + B = 1,014.2
Age in years x 4.7	= _____	= D	55 x 4.7 = 258.5
C - D	= _____	= E	C - D = 755.7

E + 655 = the number of calories you burn at rest daily: 755.7 + 655 = 1,410.7

This is a rough estimate because the calculation does not take into account individual muscle mass.

If you substitute different ages in the calculation, you will see that BMR decreases as age increases, so we'll have a tendency to put on a few pounds over the years even if we're watching what we eat and how much we're eating. Use exercise to reduce middle-age weight gain and to maintain a higher BMR. Weight training is especially good because it will help your shape by toning and strengthening your muscles and by making your body a more efficient calorie burner.

Exercise

For the midlife woman, a regular exercise program is more important than dieting to control weight gain. So, why aren't you exercising? Check all that apply.

_____ You don't have time to fit it in.

_____ You don't have access to equipment.

_____ You don't have social support/peer pressure.

_____ You don't like exercise.

_____ You don't like to sweat and be short of breath (is this really the way it's supposed to feel?).

_____ You've been smoking to control your weight.

What benefits do you want to get from exercise? And let's face it, if you're going to put this much effort into this activity, you'd better get a lot back! Check all that apply, and feel free to add some of your own.

_____ Build bone

_____ Burn calories

_____ Decrease muscle wasting and rebuild muscle mass

_____ Increase metabolic rate

_____ Improve flexibility and coordination

_____ Decrease depression

_____ Increase self-confidence

_____ Improve sleep

_____ Replace hormone therapy for menopause symptoms

_____ Redistribute body fat

_____ Slenderize your figure

_____ Control your appetite

_____ Lose weight permanently

_____ Help treat a chronic medical condition, for example, hypertension, high cholesterol, arthritis, diabetes, or urinary incontinence

_____ Reduce breast cancer risk by avoiding weight gain

_____ _____

_____ _____

_____ _____

Go back and star the three benefits that are most important to you. It will bring focus to your efforts.

I confess that I really don't like to exercise, but I love the benefits and long-term results. So I stay focused on these benefits when I'm tempted to slack off my exercise regimen. And, when building bone and muscle or improving sleep and mood isn't enough, I begin to chant, "Cruisewear, cruisewear..."

What exercises should you be doing?

Do you do any walking, dancing, hiking, jogging, or running? These are *weight-bearing exercises*. You do these at 60–80 percent of your target heart rate for best results. Target heart rate = 220 - your current age. If you are fifty, that's 220 - 50 = 170; you should be performing your weight-bearing exercises so that your heart is beating 102 to 136 times a minute. How often? Three to seven times a week.

You can determine your heart rate by finding your pulse on the side of your neck or wrist and counting the number of beats for ten seconds. If your heart rate is lower than the range listed below, speed up your activity. If your heart rate is higher than the range listed below, slow down your activity.

Here is a handy chart of target heart rates.

Age	10-second target heart rate	60-second target heart rate
20	20–27 heartbeats	120–162 heartbeats
25	20–26	120–156
30	19–25	114–150
35	19–25	114–150
40	18–24	108–144
45	18–23	108–138
50	17–23	102–138
55	17–23	102–138
60	16–22	96–132
65	16–21	96–126
70	15–20	90–120

For the greatest aerobic benefit, exercise at your target heart rate for fifteen to eighteen minutes per exercise session. Therefore, for each session, you will need a minimum of six to eight minutes to get to your target heart rate, fifteen to eighteen minutes to maintain this activity level, and six to ten minutes to cool down, or twenty-six to thirty-six minutes, total.

Do you work out with weights, use exercise machines, resistance bands, or practice Pilates techniques? These are *resistance exercises.* You must eat proteins to feed your muscles when you do these exercises. How often should you exercise? Two to three times a week.

Do you practice yoga, do stretches or isometrics? These are *balance and postural exercises*. They are great for decreasing muscle tension and improving coordination. How often? Try to do one or two of these exercises every day.

There are excellent books available that describe exercises, techniques, and tools. If you want more personalized help, trainers are good teachers and can help you learn how your body responds to exercise.

Current Concepts and Practices

For the midlife woman, a regular exercise program is more important than dieting to control weight gain. In fact, as we age, dieting becomes less and less effective in achieving weight loss, so exercise is the key.

The following is a basic Exercise Prescription:
- Weight-bearing exercises three to seven times weekly at your target heart rate
- Resistance exercises two to three times weekly (if you're really strong, add weights)
- Isometric exercises throughout the day to maintain posture and relieve tension
- Balance exercises twice daily

You *can* "spot" exercise for those pesky body areas with cellulite. Target the thighs, hips, and buttocks with resistance exercises because strengthening and toning the muscle under the superficial fat layer improves the appearance of the skin and decreases the dimpling effect.

The best exercises for midlife women are resistance exercises because they:
- Tone and strengthen your muscles
- Increase your metabolic rate
- Redistribute body fat
- Slenderize the figure
- Don't require you to severely reduce your caloric intake

Use of free weights, exercise machines, resistance bands, and Pilates techniques are all resistance-type exercises.

Weight-bearing exercises are aerobic exercises such as walking, dancing, and stair climbing (low impact); hiking, jogging, and running (high impact). These build bone by increasing bones' absorption of calcium. They burn calories efficiently if performed at your target heart rate for a minimum of eighteen minutes per exercise session.

Isometric and balance exercises such as yoga, stretching, and postural exercises increase flexibility and muscle strength and improve coordination. You only need a few minutes every day to perform these exercises.

When you're exercising regularly, you will need to eat protein. The food groups that have the highest amount of protein are meat, fish, and poultry. The second highest protein food groups are whole grains, beans, seeds, and nuts. About three ounces of protein daily—the equivalent in size and weight to a pack of playing cards—is all you'll need for "muscle food."

There is a difference between the amount of exercise you'll need to do to maintain a healthy weight and the amount you'll need to do to lose weight. It takes thirty minutes of exercise daily at moderate intensity to maintain healthy weight (that's burning from 600 to 1,200 calories a week). This thirty minutes can be broken down into smaller segments of time so that you can fit it in during the day. To lose weight, you'll have to spend more time exercising. The *Journal of the American Medical Association* recommends at least exercising three hours and fifteen minutes weekly (forty-five minutes per day, five days a week) as well as cutting back your caloric intake. To reduce your body fat by one pound, you must burn 3,500 calories. You'll need to burn about 2,800 calories a week—400 calories a day, every day, or 560 calories a day, five days a week—to lose weight at all. Fortunately, formal exercise is not the only way to burn off calories; all activity counts (but some activities count more than others).

How many calories you burn in any given activity depends on the activity and will vary with each individual because this depends on your weight and physical conditioning. The more you weigh, the more calories you will burn if you don't have too much muscle wasting.

How many calories are burned per hour of activity? The following is a list of common activities. Compare your weekly activities to these. Are you a high- or low-calorie burner? Interestingly, every one of my girlfriends performs a high calorie burning activity at least once weekly. Their ability to maintain normal body weight isn't luck, after all!

AVERAGE NUMBER OF CALORIES BURNED IN ONE HOUR OF ACTIVITY

Average Calories Burned	One Hour of
500–600	Aerobic exercise
	Stair climbing
	Running 12-minute miles
	Tennis, singles
400–500	Dancing, Jazzercise
	Hiking
	Walking 3–4 miles per hour
300–400	Cycling
	Gardening, mowing the lawn
	Moving furniture
200–300	House cleaning: mopping floors, scrubbing the bathroom, sweeping, vacuuming
	Walking the dog
	Golf

Source: American College of Sports Medicine

You don't have to exercise for months before you see any benefits. There is plenty of immediate gratification from exercise: increased confidence, reduced levels of stress, brightened mood, better sex, improved quality of sleep.

If you are thin, you will need exercise for its health benefits (protection against cancer, arthritis, bone wasting, and depression). Because you are thin, you'll need to do plenty of walking, jogging, and weight training. Your heavier counterpart is doing both aerobics and weight training every time she takes a step.

When trying to burn off calories, slow workouts and fast workouts burn about the same number of fat calories, even though the total number of calories burned is more in a faster workout than in a slow one.

Exercise can control hunger pangs and, if you don't increase your calorie intake when exercising, you'll start to burn your body fat for fuel. The good news is that we women tend to lose our stomach fat first and it feels good to have our waistbands feel loose and lie flat.

Weight training needs very little time to accomplish—thirty minutes for total body toning or ten to twelve minutes per body part, i.e., lower body, upper body, and abdominal. The standard prescription for training any body part is to do as little as one to three sets of an exercise with no more than fifteen repetitions of that exercise per set. You should take one day off between routines to rest your muscles. This will give you the best results in muscle strengthening.

If you've been sedentary throughout your adult life and you want to obtain the health benefits of exercising and/or weight loss, this is how you can start becoming a physically active person:

- Set your goals and use a log to record your physical activity and formal exercise every day. The key is to be active every day (but doesn't require a formal workout every day). You can use the forms that follow.
- You can incorporate physical activity into everyday living by dividing exercise into ten to fifteen minute segments performed throughout the day, for example, a brisk walk, housework, and gardening (remember: all physical activity counts).

- If you enjoy walking, get an inexpensive pedometer from a sporting goods store and work up to a goal of four miles per day (that's ten thousand steps as measured on the pedometer).
- If you are in an office setting most days, you can perform exercises by doing two things at once, for example, walking in place while on the phone or isometric and balance exercises between appointments.
- If you prefer using exercise equipment, put it where you will probably use it—in front of a window or the TV.

The point is to make it your goal to go from being a sedentary person to being a physically active person by committing to moving your body every day.

The website of the American College of Sports Medicine is a good place to explore to get more tips on exercise and fitness: www.acsm.org.

Combating midlife weight gain involves changing our behavior. The two most common behavior problems of overweight women are underactivity and overeating/drinking. Surveys indicate that women give the following reasons for their habit of inactivity:

- I don't have time to fit it in.
- I don't have access to exercise equipment.
- I dislike exercise because it makes me sweaty and short of breath.
- I use smoking to control my weight gain.

Eating behaviors are habits, and we women eat for comfort. We eat oversized portions, too many snack foods, and drink too much alcohol. Eating sugary carbohydrates improves our mood. We use certain carbohydrates like drugs when we're under stress. And even though we'll cut back on high-fat foods, we'll replace these calories with high-sugar foods.

How can you change behavior? Research psychologists have defined the process whereby we can successfully make behavior changes. The stages of change are:

- Intellectualizing: this is the stage where we are thinking about the problem, increasing our knowledge, and assessing our benefits and risks.
- Committing: at this stage, we are ready for change and have made a commitment to ourselves. During this stage, we consider using social supports, define the behaviors we want to change, and we fantasize about rewarding ourselves for achieving our goals.
- Planning: this involves developing a plan of action that requires that we identify at least two personal benefits of change. We select enjoyable activities and a specific time and place for these activities, and we outline a plan.
- Action: in this final stage, we contract with ourselves to carry out a plan that identifies our roadblocks and risks for relapse and that has defined time limits and rewards. We put the plan into action with the help of our social supports.

You can lose weight at any age but, as you age, this is going to involve changing your lifestyle. With some experimentation and patience, you can get results. And remember, exercise is the foundation of your weight-loss program, not dieting.

GOAL SHEET

Goals are things a person really wants to do. They add an element of balance to life.

_____ Today's Weight   _____ Goal Weight

List three reasons why you want to reach your goal.

1. _____
2. _____
3. _____

Identify two people who will support you in a healthy lifestyle.

1. _____
2. _____

Picture yourself having attained your goal weight—what you want to be doing, how you want to feel—and hold on to that mental picture. Remember: your journey of a thousand miles begins with a single step. Record those steps on the Exercise Log that follows. And good luck!

Log your weight at:

_____ 6 weeks   _____ 9 months
_____ 3 months   _____ 1 year
_____ 6 months   _____ 2 years

Exercise Log

My Goal: _____

Sunday	Monday	Tuesday	Wednesday	Total

Exercise Log

My Goal: _____

Thursday	Friday	Saturday	Total

Chapter 37

A Reference Guide
to Improving Your Health

The manufacture and sale of vitamins and supplements is a billion-dollar industry. Many of you are trying these treatments because of unsubstantiated claims of cures based on limited research. In fact, most of the information about the effectiveness of these treatments is coming from magazines and user promotions, not research. Be cautious in your use of supplements.

A major cause of illness among prescription medication users is drug-to-drug interaction. This same problem can and will occur with supplement use. I've experienced adverse interactions, myself.

Please use this chapter carefully as a reference. *These are incompletely researched and unproven recommendations. Many are now being researched because of claims of effectiveness. Specifically, their short-term and long-term effects have not yet been clearly demonstrated, nor have their interactions.*

This is how to use this chapter:

- Choose conditions that are of interest to you.
- If you have multiple medical problems, focus on one at a time.
- Discuss these recommendations with your doctor and decide which ones will be safe to try.
- Follow your doctor's advice about diet changes, supplement dosages, and exercise limits.

More is not better. The supplements mentioned are reported as individually effective, so within any one category of problem, do not consume more than one or two supplements at the same time. Avoid using products with multiple, combined supplements except for multivitamins. Most good multivitamins will give you adequate, recommended dosages of vitamins and minerals.

Please notice that there are many recommendations in common across these categories of medical conditions, and making changes under one medical problem can be useful in prevention of others.

The following is a list of medical problems that can occur in the postmenopausal years:

- Wrinkles and cellulite accumulation
- High cholesterol
- High blood pressure
- Obesity
- Urinary tract disorders
- Sexual dysfunction
- Diabetes
- Heart disease
- Osteoporosis
- Arthritis
- Depression
- Cancer
- Alzheimer's disease

QUIZ

Do you have any of these conditions? If so, list them:

_____

Are you at risk for any of these conditions? If so, list them:

_____

Are you taking prescription medications, vitamins, or over-the-counter drugs? If so, list them:

_____

Let's see what's useful for the following conditions or problems.

WRINKLES AND CELLULITE
(Aging skin and fat accumulation under the skin)

Diet – Follow one that's high in fruits, vegetables, fish, olive oil, beans, and water, and low in animal fats and dairy. Avoid caffeine and sugar. Don't smoke. Use sunscreen outdoors.

Dietary supplements – Useful vitamins are A, C, and E. Useful herbs are green tea, gingko biloba, grape seed, sweet clover, and evening primrose oil. Remember: no more than one or two at a time.

Exercise – Best choice: lower body weight training. Second choice: daily aerobics of moderate intensity.

High Cholesterol
(High blood serum cholesterol)

Diet – Follow one high in mono- and polyunsaturated fats (like fish and olive oil) and low in meat and dairy. Substitute for margarine and salad dressings (try Benecol or Take Control). Avoid dietary cholesterol.

Habits – Don't smoke.

Supplements – Useful are soy protein, omega-3 fatty acids, fiber, garlic, and flaxseed.

Exercise – Best choice: walking two hours a day. Second choice: running or jogging twenty miles a week.

High Blood Pressure
(Greater than 140/90)

Diet – The DASH diet (Dietary Approaches to Stop Hypertension) is high in fruits, vegetables, and whole grains, and low in animal fat, dairy, dietary cholesterol (less than 200 mg daily), and salt (less than one teaspoonful daily). Avoid processed foods and alcohol. Eliminate caffeine.

Supplements – Useful minerals are calcium, magnesium, and potassium. Also useful are phytoestrogens, especially soy protein.

Exercise – Best choice: walking daily for about thirty-five to forty minutes, or about two miles (low and moderate intensity). Second choice: all forms of physical activity, for example, gardening, if done regularly.

Obesity
(BMI greater than 30; see chapters 35 & 36)

Diet – No single diet is right for all women. You must reduce the total number of calories you consume daily. Eliminate starch, sugar, and alcohol.

Supplements – Useful minerals are calcium, magnesium, and chromium. Useful prescription drugs are Meridia and Xenical. These must be prescribed by a doctor and must always be used with diet and exercise.

Exercise – Your weight loss goal is one to two pounds a week. Best choice: muscle toning and strengthening two to three times a week. Second choice: aerobics daily.

Urinary Tract Disorders
(Urinary incontinence and recurrent infections)

Diet – To treat infections, eat plain yogurt and drink unsweetened cranberry juice and plenty of water. Follow a diet low in starches and sugars. Eliminate caffeine and alcohol.

Habits – Stop smoking.

Supplements – Useful are acidophilus and vitamin C.

Exercise – Try Kegel exercises daily for incontinence. A good exercise program for weight control can be found in chapter 36.

Sexual Dysfunction
(Vaginal dryness and decreased libido)

Diet – Follow one high in whole soy food, for example, soybeans and tofu.

Supplements – L-arginine, vitamin E, niacin, ginseng, and gingko biloba are useful, as are topical lubricants and vitamin E suppositories.

Phytoestrogens – Useful are black cohosh, dandelion leaves, oat straw, wild yam, dong quai, and chasteberry.

Exercise – All types help.

Diabetes
(Type II)

Diet – The USDA Pyramid Diet is harmful. It recommends consuming too many carbohydrates, doesn't differentiate between high-quality carbs and low-quality carbs, and recommends too much dairy. Follow one high in complex carbohydrates, fiber, vegetables, whole grains, beans, monounsaturated fats, omega-3 fatty acids, and drink plenty of water. Follow one low in fruits, nuts, and dairy. Eliminate starches, sugars, and "below-ground" carbohydrates, such as potatoes.

Habits — Switch to artificial sweeteners.

Supplements — Use multivitamins with chromium, magnesium, and selenium. Useful vitamins are A, C, E, and folic acid, though vitamin E may interfere with absorption of your diabetic medication. Check with your doctor. Also useful is flaxseed.

Exercise — Weight reduction is important. Your exercise plan should include muscle strengthening two times a week and aerobics three times a week. Insulin is a growth hormone; abnormally low levels will lead to muscle wasting. Certain diabetic medications are also muscle wasting, as are the statins often used to treat diabetics for high or potentially high cholesterol.

Heart Disease
(Coronary artery disease)

Diet — Follow one high in whole grains, complex carbohydrates, fiber, vegetables, fish, and poultry, and low in fats (less than 30 percent of your daily calories), low in cholesterol (less than 300 mg daily), low in meat, butter, and dairy products. Avoid salt and alcohol. Eliminate fast foods.

Habits — Stop smoking. Take one low dose aspirin daily.

Supplements — Useful vitamins are A, C, E, folic acid, B6, and B12; also useful are magnesium, coenzyme Q, garlic, and omega-3 fatty acids.

Exercise — Best choice: walking, either vigorous or moderate, at least one hour daily. The longer you walk, the more preventive is the exercise.

Osteoporosis and Osteopenia

Diet – Follow one high in low-fat dairy products, cold-water fish, lean meat, poultry, beans, whole grains, and dark green leafy vegetables, and low in salt. Avoid soda, caffeine, and alcohol.

Habits – Stop smoking.

Supplements – Use calcium, magnesium, and vitamin D.

Phytoestrogens – Use soy protein and green tea.

Exercise – Best choice: weight training.

Arthritis
(Osteoarthritis)

Diet – Follow one high in vegetables, cold-water fish, apples, berries, and water. Drink half your body weight in ounces of water daily (if you weigh 160 pounds, drink 80 ounces of water every day). Cook with olive oil and flaxseed oil. Eliminate fast foods, microwave entrees, fried foods, bakery goods, and margarine.

Supplements – Useful are vitamins C, D, and E, omega-3 and omega-6 fatty acids, and selenium. Other useful supplements are kava (for muscle ache and spasm), glucosamine (1,500 mg daily), and chondroitin (1,200 mg daily) for pain (remember: take one or two at a time), and basil, oregano, and garlic seasonings.

Exercise – Best choice: stretching, for example, yoga. Second choice: muscle strengthening and low-impact aerobics.

Depression and Anxiety

Diet – Follow one high in vegetables, fruit, whole grains, low-fat dairy products, fish, lean meat, and poultry. Avoid sugar, flour, saturated fats, and caffeine — while these elevate brain serotonin (and lift mood), they cause weight gain. Eliminate alcohol; it has addictive potential due to the temporary relief it provides.

Supplements – For mild to moderate symptoms, use kava, passion flower, valerian, St. John's wort, GABA, or SAMe. Remember: one or two at a time, as always.

Exercise – Best choice: aerobics daily (moderate to intense).

Cancer
(Lung, breast, colon, uterus)

Diet – Follow one high in green vegetables, fruits, whole grains, and beans, and low in animal proteins and saturated fats. Avoid alcohol.

Habits – Stop smoking. Minimize weight gain. Taking one baby aspirin daily is useful for colon cancer.

Supplements – Useful vitamins and minerals are vitamins A, C, and E, folic acid, calcium, magnesium, and selenium. Other useful supplements are flaxseed, green tea, and garlic.

Exercise – Best choice: aerobics of moderate intensity, at least four hours/week.

Alzheimer's Disease

Diet – Follow one high in green leafy vegetables, fruits, whole grains, and fish, and low in saturated fats.

Habits – Get mental exercise. Read, do crossword puzzles, play cards. I know you'll remember this, it's not a new thought: use it or lose it!

Supplements – Useful vitamins are E, folic acid, B6, B12, and C; useful minerals are zinc and selenium. Other useful supplements include choline, coenzyme Q10, aspirin, such amino acids as tyrosine and glutamine, and herbs like gingko biloba and ginseng.

Exercise – Engage in daily physical activity of all types.

Chapter 38

The SANE Approach to Developing Your MAP

In 1999, I founded a company called Women's HealthSource whose mission is to educate women about midlife health. I developed and we conduct wellness workshops for business as well as a series of seminars open to all. These seminars provide women with an opportunity to obtain the information they seek from a medical professional, to explore their options with other women who can understand their experiences, and to better prepare themselves to discuss their midlife health issues with their doctors. Each program brings together small groups of women who have questions to ask, experiences to share, a concern for their present and future health, and a common interest in becoming informed healthcare consumers.

This book has evolved from the discussions I've had with these groups of women. The issues we struggled with are those I've researched and discussed in this book. The information and exercises in parts I through IV have been designed to prepare you for part V, and part V has been about what you can do for yourself to foster a happy, healthy change of life.

There are a few basic principles I'd like you to remember and commit yourself to. I call them the SANE approach to disease prevention and health maintenance.

The SANE Approach

S — Stop smoking.

A — Avoid alcohol.

N — Nourish your body with good nutrition; vitamin supplements are a must.

E — Exercise daily, just as you brush your teeth and go to work daily.

We are the Baby Boomers and we are entering our maturity. We are:

• Making an effort to find ways to stay healthy as long as we can;

• Getting the tools and guidance we need from our medical experts;

• Learning ways to slow the aging process through lifestyle changes and better nutrition; and

• Wanting and willing to help ourselves rather than relying solely on other authorities.

Let's turn to completing your MAP now.

Part VI

The MAP

Chapter 39

Completing the
Menopause Action Plan

The MAP is a set of worksheets that will help you define your problems, identify your health concerns, and formulate solutions to them. The screening tests and risk assessments in this book are a kind of early warning system also designed to help you complete the MAP. Ideally, you will complete part I of the MAP after completing part I of the book, part II of the MAP after part II of the book, part III after part III, etc. Not only will the material be fresher than if you do it all at one time, but the effort won't seem so daunting. In any event, should you draw a blank or become confused while answering one of the questions on the MAP, go back to the corresponding part of the book and look for the answer.

Your MAP is the product of your reading and thinking. It identifies the issues that are relevant to you. You have some very good ideas about how you can live a healthy life and a lot to talk about with your doctor. Go to it: I encourage you to take a greater part in actively managing you own menopause and your own future health. The best of health to you!

Chapter 40

Part I—My Current Symptoms

What are your most bothersome change of life symptoms?
List them:
Did you have PMS during puberty or during the young-adult years? If so, list your symptoms: _____

_____

_____

Attach a copy of the screening examinations appropriate for your decade (see part II, chapter 10).

Chapter 41

Part II — My Medical History

Circle the term that best fits the group of symptoms you are
  experiencing.
  PMS   Perimenopause   Menopause   Postmenopause   None
List the medical/psychiatric conditions for which you are
  currently being treated: _____

_____

List your current habits (for example, smoking, drinking,
  recreational drug use):_____
Do you have a history of problems in: If so, describe them:
  Pre-Puberty _____
  Menarche _____
  Childbearing Years _____
  Midlife _____
  Older Adult Years

  _____

Most recent test/measurement results:
  Blood pressure _____
  Pulse rate _____
  Height _____
  Weight _____

List all your current prescription medications and their dosages:

_____

List all nonprescription drugs you are taking, including vitamins
and minerals:

_____

Have you had the following tests within the past twelve months?
    If so, record the results:
    Pelvic exam and PAP smear   Yes   No _____
    Mammography   Yes   No _____
    Blood glucose   Yes   No _____
    Lipid profile (total cholesterol, LDL, HDL, triglycerides)
        Yes   No _____
    Urinalysis   Yes   No _____
    Follicle-stimulating hormone   Yes   No _____
    Thyroid-stimulating hormone   Yes   No _____
    Bone mineral density   Yes   No _____

Chapter 42

Part III — Disease Risks

Which diseases do you worry about getting? List them:

_____

List those diseases for which you are at risk:

_____

Are you having any early signs or symptoms of disease?
   Which disease(s)? _____

Do the diseases you have listed above have any risk factors
   in common?   Yes   No

If yes, list them: _____

Can any of these risks be changed?   Yes   No

If yes, which risk factors are you willing to work on? List them:

_____

My **first commitment** is to schedule an appointment with my
   doctor for further evaluation.
   My doctor's name is:

_____

Address:

_____

Phone:

_____

My appointment is scheduled for:

_____

Date:

_____

Time:

_____

Chapter 43

Part IV—HRT Assessment

Quiz

I have decided to try HRT. Circle one.   Yes   No

If yes, continue. If no, proceed to the table listing alternative treatments.

I am currently taking HRT and have decided to continue with it.
     Yes   No

I know I can take HRT safely because I have discussed it with
     my doctor.   Yes   No

I have completed my Disease Risk Assessments and have had the
     laboratory tests and examinations recommended for my age.
     Yes   No

I have no contraindications to taking HRT.   Yes   No

My reasons for taking HRT are (check all that apply):

_____ to get symptom relief

_____ to minimize any physical changes

_____ to obtain long-term disease protection

I am taking the following product: _____

It contains estrogen alone.   Yes   No

It contains estrogen along with progestin/progesterone.   Yes   No

   I take it: _____ orally   _____ topically   _____ vaginally

Are you getting the therapeutic benefits you hoped for?   Yes   No

My **second commitment** is to do the following when I take HRT:

- I will take HRT for no more than five years,

Or

- I have been taking HRT for more than five years and I will faithfully get all my screening examinations and laboratory tests done yearly.
- I will try alternative therapies to eventually substitute for my use of HRT.
- I will use HRT in combination with healthy eating habits and exercise.
- I will check regularly for changes in my:

    Weight

    Blood pressure

    Cholesterol

    Breasts

    I will report any side effects/changes to my doctor.

Please sign your name to this commitment:

_____ Date: _____

ALTERNATIVE TREATMENTS

If you are trying alternatives, list each product you are using, the reason for using it (indication), and its benefit to you.

Product/Medication	Indication	Benefit	No Change

Chapter 44

Part V—My Lifestyle

I prefer to change my lifestyle and habits.

Quiz

My current health problems are (from part I):

_____

My future health risks are (from part III):

_____

Habits to change (circle each number that applies):
1. Smoking—Which smoking cessation method are you going to use? _____
   When do you plan to stop? _____
2. Alcohol—By how much will you decrease your intake?

   _____
3. Lack of physical activity
4. Weight gain
5. Overeating

Eating Plan

1. How many calories do you need daily to maintain a healthy weight? _____

   Describe your eating plan for weight control, for example, pyramid, self-designed (see chapter 38).

   _____

Vitamins and Minerals

List those supplements you will add to provide your daily requirements: _____   _____

_____   _____

_____   _____

_____   _____

_____   _____

_____   _____

List those supplements you will add to provide for disease prevention (two only): _____   _____

Phytoestrogens

List those you will take for symptom relief: _____

_____   _____   _____

Weight Control

My current body mass index is: _____

My ideal BMI is between 19 and 24.

My ideal weight range is between _____and _____. These weights correspond to a BMI of 19 and a BMI of 24, for a woman of my height.

My exercise plan calls for:

_____

My diet plan calls for (type of diet, for example, pyramid, self-designed): _____

How many calories do I need daily to maintain a healthy weight? _____

At a recommended weight loss of one to two pounds per week, how many weeks will it take me to reach a BMI of 24 or less? _____

How much weight will I lose in that time? _____

My **third commitment** is to work toward disease prevention and health maintenance using the SANE approach. I will:

S — Stop smoking.

A — Avoid alcohol.

N — Nourish my body with good nutrition; vitamin supplements are a must.

E — Exercise daily, just as I brush my teeth and go to work daily.

Please sign your name to this commitment:

_____ Date: _____

Afterword

The individual is the context.

Consider carefully the forty or so years ahead of you. How well you prepare for the second half of life may be the most important decision you will ever make. As we age, good health and vitality depend on what we do to prevent problems. A good health program can be developed at any age if we have information. We will all live longer than our mothers, but without good health, that longer life is just a shadow existence. This book is my effort to answer the midlife woman's question, "What's happening to me and what does it mean?" I have filled this book with questions and exercises to make the information personally relevant to you. Most of the questions were designed to get you thinking about making changes. Change is hard but possible if you have a plan, make your steps small, and take them one at a time. There isn't any one health plan for success that can be applied to every woman. There is only *your* health plan, and you'll have to discover one for yourself through (guided) trial and error. This is the rest of your life we're talking about, so be patient and persevere. The best advice I can give you is to take personal responsibility for yourself; make habit and lifestyle changes that are proactive and preventive.

Good health and good living.

Resources

Part I
BOOKS AND ARTICLES

A Clinician's Guide to Menopause. Stewart, MD, and Robinson, MD, 1997, American Psychiatric Press, Washington, D.C.

Dr. Susan Lark's Premenstrual Syndrome Self-Help Book: A Woman's Guide to Feeling Good All Month. Susan M. Lark, MD, 1993, Celestial Arts, Berkeley, CA.

Dr. Susan Love's Menopause and Hormone Book: Making Informed Choices. Susan Love, 1997, Random House, New York, NY.

"Making Sense of Menopause." *U.S.News & World Report*, November 18, 2002.

Menopausal Years, The Wise Woman Way: Alternative Approaches for Women 30–90. Susan Weed, 1992, Ashtree Publishing, Woodstock, NY.

The Pause: Positive Approaches to Perimenopause and Menopause. Lonnie Barbach, 1993, Signet, New York, NY.

PMS Relief: Natural Approaches to Treating Symptoms. Judy E. Marshel, and Anne Egan, 1998, Berkeley Publishing Group, New York, NY.

Premenstrual Syndrome: How You Can Benefit From Diet, Vitamins, Minerals, Herbs, and Other Natural Methods. Michael T. Murray, 1997, Prima, Rocklin, CA.

The Silent Passage. Gail Sheehy, 1998, Simon & Schuster, New York, NY.

What Your Doctor May Not Tell You About Menopause: The Breakthrough Book on Natural Progesterone. John R. Lee, MD, and Hopkins, 1996, Warner Books, New York, NY.

The Wisdom of Menopause. Christiane Northrup, MD, 2001, Bantam Books, New York, NY.

A Woman Doctor's Guide to Menopause: Essential Facts and Up-to-the-Minute Information for a Woman's Change of Life. L. Jovanovic, MD, and S. Levert, 1993, Hyperion Press, New York, NY.

Women's Bodies, Women's Wisdom. Christiane Northrup, MD, 1994, Bantam Books, New York, NY.

WEBSITES

National Heart, Lung, and Blood Institute: www.nhlbi.nih.gov

North American Menopause Society: www.menopause.org

Power-surge (A virtual community for women in the pause): http://www.dearest.com

Part II
Books and Articles

Our Bodies, Ourselves for the New Century. The Boston Women's Health Book Collective, 1998, Touchstone, New York, NY.

Perimenopause. J. Huston, MD, and D. Lanka, MD, 1997, New Harbinger Publications, Oakland, CA.

The Thyroid Guide. Ditkoff, MD, and Gerfo, MD, 2000, Harper Perennial, Toronto, Ontario, Canada.

Women's Moods: What Every Woman Must Know About Hormones, the Brain, and Emotional Health. D. Sichel, MD, and J. Driscoll, 1999, William Morrow & Company, Toronto, Ontario, Canada.

Websites

Harvard Women's Health Watch: www.med.harvard.edu
Medscape, Women's Health: www.medscape.com
National Women's Health Resource Center: www.healthywomen.org

Part III
Books and Articles

Anger at Work: Learning the Art of Anger Management on the Job. H. Weisinger, PhD, 1995, William Morrow & Co., Toronto, Ontario, Canada.

Anxiety and Depression: A Natural Approach. S. Trickett, 1995, Ulysses Press, Berkeley, CA.

Anxiety and Phobia Workbook. E.J. Bourne, 2000, New Harbinger Publications, Oakland, CA.

Anxiety, Phobias, and Panic: A Step-by-Step Program for Regaining Control of Your Life. R.Z. Peurifoy, 1988, Warner Books, New York, NY.

Cancer Sourcebook for Women. K. Bellinir, Ed., 2002, Omnigraphics, Detroit, MI.

Career Success/Personal Success: How to Stay Healthy in a High-Stress Environment. C.A. Leatz, 1992, McGraw Hill, Berkeley, CA.

Dear Job Stressed: Answers for the Overworked, Overwrought, and Overwhelmed. T. Tihista, and M.H. Dempsey, 1996, Consulting Psychologists Press, San Francisco, CA.

The Depression Workbook: A Guide for Living with Depression and Manic Depression. M. Copeland, 1992, New Harbinger Publications, Oakland, CA.

Don't Panic: Taking Control of Anxiety Attacks. R. Wilson, 1996, HarperCollins, Toronto, Ontario, Canada.

How You Can Survive When They're Depressed. A. Sheffield, 1999, Random House, New York, NY.

The Osteoporosis Handbook. S. Bonnick, MD, 2001, Taylor Publishing, Dallas, TX.

Overcoming Depression. D. Papolos, 1988, Harper Collins, Toronto, Ontario, Canada.

Overcoming Panic, Anxiety, and Phobias: New Strategies to Free Yourself from Worry and Fear. C. Goodman, 1996, Whole Person Associates, Duluth, MN.

Preventing Arthritis: A Holistic Approach to Life Without Pain. Lawrence, and Zucker, 2001, Berkley Publishing Group, New York, NY.

The Relaxation and Stress Reduction Workbook. Davis, Eshelman, and McKay, 1988, New Harbinger Publications, Oakland, CA.

The Relaxation and Stress Reduction Workbook (4th Edition). Davis, Eshelman, and McKay, 1998, New Harbinger Publications, Oakland, CA.

Strong Women and Men Beat Arthritis. E. Miriam, Nelson, et al, 2002, Putnam, New York, NY.

The Thyroid Guide. Koff, and LoGerfo, MD, 2000, Harper Publishers, Toronto, Ontario, Canada.

Treatment of the Postmenopausal Woman. G.I. Gorodeski, and W.H. Ution, 1999, Lippincott, Williams, and Wilkins, Baltimore, MD.

Understanding Depression. J. DePaulo, and L. Horvitz, 1996, Wiley & Sons, Hoboken, NJ.

Undoing Depression: What Therapy Doesn't Teach You and Medication Can't Give You. R. O'Connor, 1997, Berkeley Publishing Group, New York, NY.

What the Blues Tell Us All About: Black Women Overcoming Stress and Depression. A. Mitchell, 1998, Perigee, New York, NY.

When Words Are Not Enough: The Women's Prescription for Depression and Anxiety. V. Raskin, 1997, Broadway Books, New York, NY.

WEBSITES

Alzheimer's Association: www.alz.org

American Diabetes Association: www.diabetes.org

American Thyroid Association: www.thyroid.org

Arthritis Foundation: www.arthritis.org

Dana Foundation: www.dana.org

Journal of the American Medical Association: www.ama-assn.org

Medscape, Women's Health: www.medscape.com

National Institute of Mental Health: www.nimh.nih.gov

National Institutes of Health: www.nih.gov/health/infoline.htm

National Mental Health Association (NMHA): www.nmha.org

National Osteoporosis Foundation: www.nof.org

National Stroke Association: www.stroke.org

Oncolink—University of Pennsylvania Cancer Center: www.oncolink.com

Prevention Magazine: www.prevention.com

U.S. Department of Health and Human Services: www.healthfinder.gov

Woman's Diagnostic Cyber News: www.wdxcyber.com/nmood.htm#pms

Women's Heart Foundation: www.womensheart.org

Part IV
BOOKS AND ARTICLES

"Diet, Phytoestrogens, and Prevention of Breast Cancer." *Menopause: The Journal of the North American Menopause Society (NAMS)*, vol. 2, 2000.

Estrogen: A Complete Guide to Menopause and Hormone Replacement Therapy (3rd Edition). E. Nachtigal, MD, and J. Heilman, 2000, HarperCollins Publishers, Toronto, Ontario, Canada.

"Evaluating ERT/HRT for Postmenopausal Women." *Menopause Management*, vol. 10, January, 2001.

Managing Menopause with Diet and Herbs. L. Beck, RD, 2000, Prentice Hall, Toronto, Ontario, Canada.

The Osteoporosis Handbook: Every Woman's Guide to Prevention and Treatment (3rd Edition). S. Bonnick, MD, FACP, 2001, Taylor Publishing, Dallas, TX.

The Wisdom of Menopause. Northrup, MD, 2001, Bantam Books, New York, NY.

A Woman Doctor's Guide to Menopause. Javanovic, MD, and Levert, 1993, Hyperion Press, New York, NY.

Women's Encyclopedia of Natural Medicine: Alternative Therapies and Integrative Medicine. T. Hudson, ND, 1999, Keats Publishing, Los Angeles, CA.

Women's Moods: What Every Woman Must Know about Hormones, the Brain, and Emotional Health. D. Sichel, MD, and J. Driscoll, MS/RN/CS, 1999, William Morrow & Co., New York, NY.

NEWSLETTERS

Harvard Women's Health Watch
P.O. Box 420068
Palm Cost, FL 32142
Toll Free U.S./Canada 800-829-5921
Outside U.S./Canada 904-445-4662
www.med.harvard.edu

HerbalGram
American Botanical Council
P.O. Box 144345
Austin, TX 78714
Toll Free U.S./Canada 800-373-7105
Outside U.S./Canada 512-331-8868
www.herbalgram.org

The Soy Connection
Communiqué, Inc.
P.O. Box 237
Jefferson City, MO 65102
573-635-3265
www.talksoy.com

Tufts University Health & Nutrition Letter: Your Guide to Living Healthier, Longer
Tufts University
P.O. Box 420235
Palm Coast, FL 32142
Toll Free U.S./Canada 800-274-7581
Outside U.S./Canada 617-350-7994
www.healthletter.tufts.edu

WEBSITES
Journal of the American Medical Association: www.ama-assn.org
National Women's Health Network: Taking Hormones and Women's Health; www.womenshealthnetwork.org
National Women's Health Resource Center: www.healthywomen.org
North American Menopause Society: www.menopause.org

Part V
BOOKS AND ARTICLES
The American Pharmaceutical Association Practical Guide to Natural Medicines. Pierce, Gans, and Weil, 1999, William Morrow & Co., Toronto, Ontario, Canada.
Callanetics Fit Forever. C. Pinckney, 1995, Perigee Press, New York, NY.
The Carbohydrate Addict's Diet. Rachael Heller, and Richard Heller, 1993, Signet, New York, NY.
Complete Guide to Exercise Videos. Collage Video catalog updated regularly. 800-433-6769.
The DASH Diet for Hypertension. Moor, MD, and Svetkey, MD, 2002, Simon & Shuster, New York, NY.
Definition. J. Vedral, PhD, 1995, Warner Books, New York, NY.
Dietary Reference Intakes. Institute of Medicine Standing Committee on Scientific Evaluation of Dietary Intakes, 1997, National Academy Press, Washington, D.C.
Dr. Atkins' New Diet Revolution. R. Atkins, MD, 1992, Avon Books, Toronto, Ontario, Canada.
Enter The Zone. B. Sears, 1995, HarperCollins Publishers, New York, NY.

Estrogen, The Natural Way. N. Shandler, 2000, Villard Press, New York, NY.

The Fitness Factor. L. Callahan, 2002, Lyons Press, Guilford, CT.

Herbal Medicine: Expanded Commission and Monographs. Blumenthal, and Goldberg, 2000, Integrative Medicine Communications, Newton, MA.

Herbal Medicines. C. Fetrow, and J. Avila, 2000, Pocket Books, New York, NY.

Herbal Medicines. Expert Committee of the German Federal Institute for Drugs, 2000, Integrative Medicine Communications, Newton, MA.

Herbal Medicines. Newall, Anderson, and Phillipson, 1996, Pharmaceutical Press, London, England.

Herbs of Choice. V. Taylor, 1998, Haworth Press, Binghamton, NY.

Keep Your Brain Young. McKhann, MD, and Albert, PhD, 2002, Wiley & Sons, Hoboken, NJ.

Managing Menopause with Diet and Herbs. L. Beck, RD, 2000, Prentice Hall, Toronto, Ontario, Canada.

Menopause and Homeopathy. I. Kenge, and A. Kenge, 1999, North Atlantic Books, Berkeley, CA.

Outsmarting the Midlife Fat Cell. D. Waterhouse, 1998, Hyperion, New York, NY.

A Path to Healing: A Guide to Wellness. A. Sullivan, PhD, 2001, Doubleday, New York, NY.

PDR for Herbal Medicines. 1998, Medical Economics Co., Montvale, NJ.

Preventing Arthritis. R. Lawrence, MD, S. Andrews, MD, and L. Balart, MD, 1998, Ballantine Publishing Group, New York, NY.

Protein Power. Michael Eades, and Mary Eades, 1996, Bantam, New York, NY.

Real-World Fitness. K. Kaehler, 1999, Golden Books Adult Publishing, New York, NY.

Strength Book. J. Wharton, and P. Wharton, 1999, Random House, New York, NY.

Strong Women Stay Young. M. Nelson, PhD, and S. Wernick, 2000, Bantam Books, New York, NY.

Strong Women Stay Young (Revised Edition). Wilson, Wray, and Wernick, 2000, Bantam Books, New York, NY.

Sugarbusters. Stewart, MD, Bethea, MD, and Andrews, MD, 1998, Ballantine Publishing, New York, NY.

The Vitamins. G. Combs, 1991, Academic Press, London, England.

Women's Encyclopedia of Natural Medicine: Alternative Therapies and Integrative Medicine. T. Hudson, 1999, Keats Publishing, Los Angeles, CA.

Women's Moods. D. Sichel, MD, 1999, William Morrow & Co., Toronto, Ontario, Canada.

Women, Weight, and Hormones. E. Vhet, 2001, Evans & Co., New York, NY.

WEBSITES

About: Health and Fitness: www.about.com/health

American Council on Exercise: www.acefitness.org/fitfacts

As We Change (product ordering magazine for midlife women): www.aswechange.com

Columbia University and Rosenthal Center: http://cpmcnet. columbia.edu/dept/rosenthal

Dr. Andrew Weil's Web Page: www.drweil.com

eDiets: www.ediets.com

Harvard's *Women's Health Watch*: www.med.harvard.edu

HerbalGram: www.herbalgram.org

National Council on Alcoholism: www.ncadd.org

National Institute of Aging (NIA): www.nia.nih.gov

National Institute of Health Office of Alternative Medicine (OAM): http://altmed.od.nih.gov

Puritan's Pride: www.puritan.com

Solo Fitness, Inc.: www.solofitness.com

Sports Music: www.workoutmusicvideo.com

Tufts University Health & Nutrition Letter: www.healthletter. tufts.edu

U.S. Department of Agriculture: www.nal.usda.gov

Index

About the Author

Marsha Lynn Speller, MD, is the founder and Executive Director of Women's HealthSource, Inc., which offers Change of Life seminars to women and women's midlife health education programs to businesses. She is a certified menopause clinician and participates in clinical research pertaining to menopause symptoms and treatment. She exclusively sees women in her private practice and believes psychiatry truly is the study of women across the life cycle. She conducts a free spring lecture series on the health issues of midlife women and is a guest columnist for her community newspaper.

Dr. Speller grew up in the Philadelphia area, the daughter of two physicians. She is a graduate of Howard University Medical School and completed her specialty training in psychiatry at New York State Psychiatric Institute (Columbia University) and McLean Hospital (Harvard University). She returned to the Philadelphia area to start a family and taught at Thomas Jefferson University in the Department of Psychiatry for several years. She still lives in the Delaware Valley with her husband and two college-age children.